Teens,
Tattoos, & Piercings

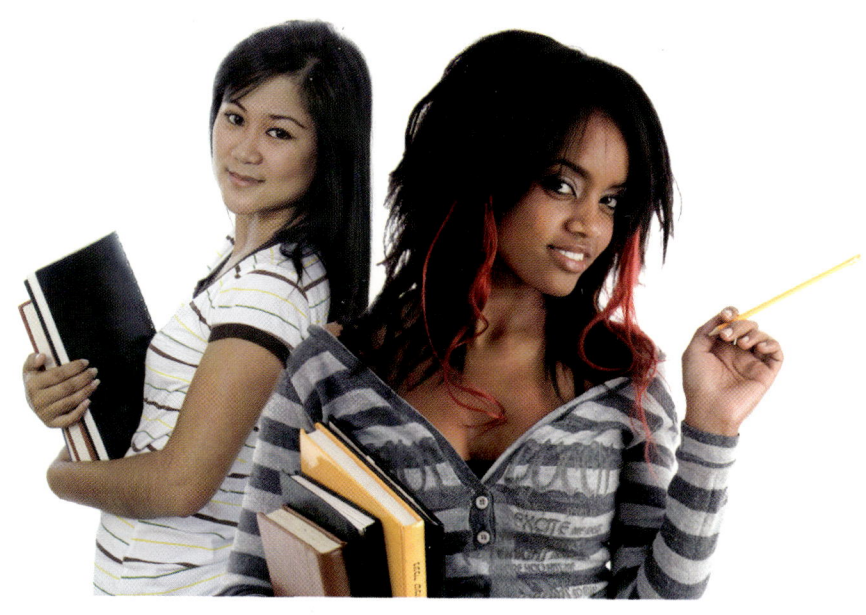

The health & social impact of permanent body art.

Gregory L. Hall, MD

Teens, Tattoos, & Piercings
The health & social impact of permanent body art.

First Edition
Copyright © 2012 by Integrative Clinical Resources, Inc.

ISBN-13: 978-0-9858587-0-4 (Gregory Hall, MD)
ISBN-10: 0985858702

Printed in the United States of America
First Printing: July 2012
Second Printing: October 2012

Warning and Disclaimer

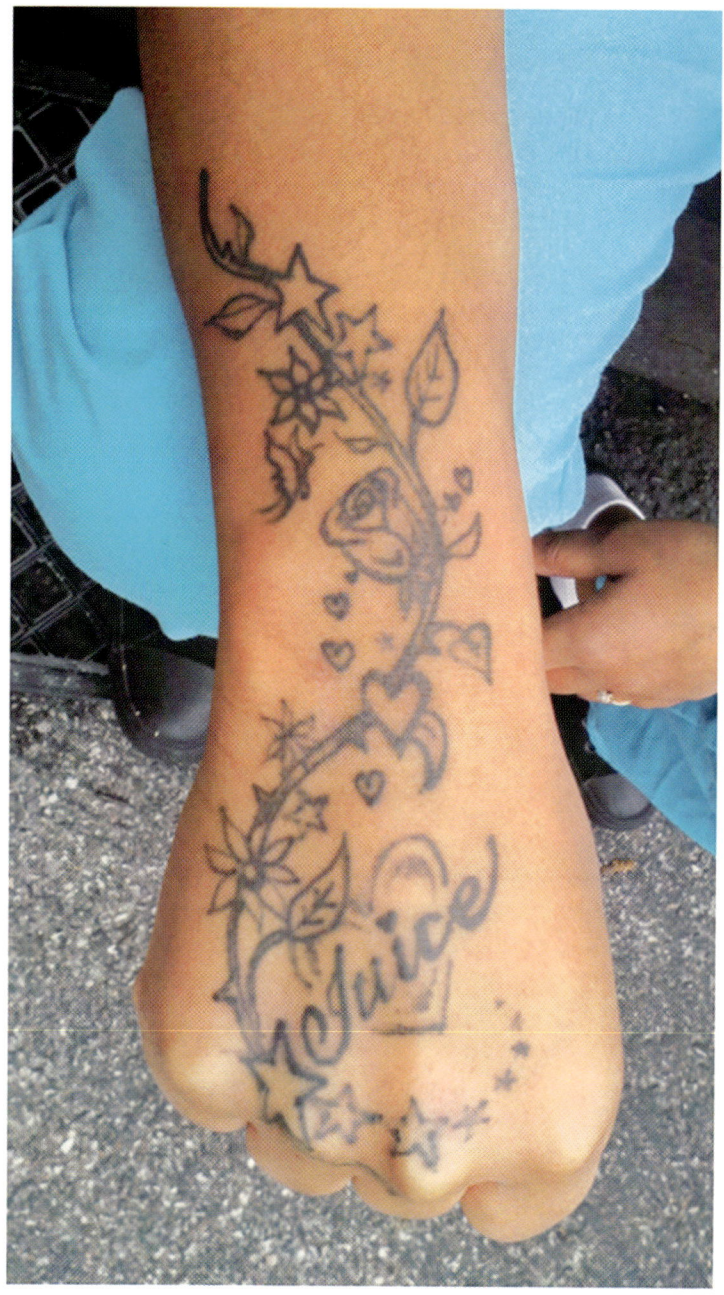

Bulk Sales

Integrative Clinical Resources offers *significant discounts* on this book when ordered in quantity for bulk purchases or special sales. Because of these discounts, schools and organizations have conducted fund raising book sales that have resulted in significant revenue for their cause.

Call to find out how your organization can get good information to teens, and improve its revenue.

For more information please contact:
Integrative Clinical Resources, LLC
464 Richmond Road
Suite 201
Richmond Heights, Ohio 44143
216 881-5055

**For more up to date information,
Go to
TeensTattoosAndPiercings.com**

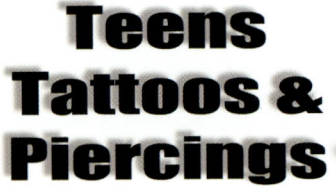 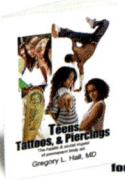 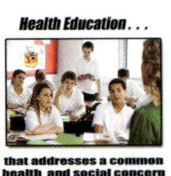 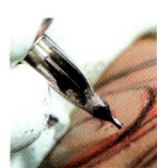

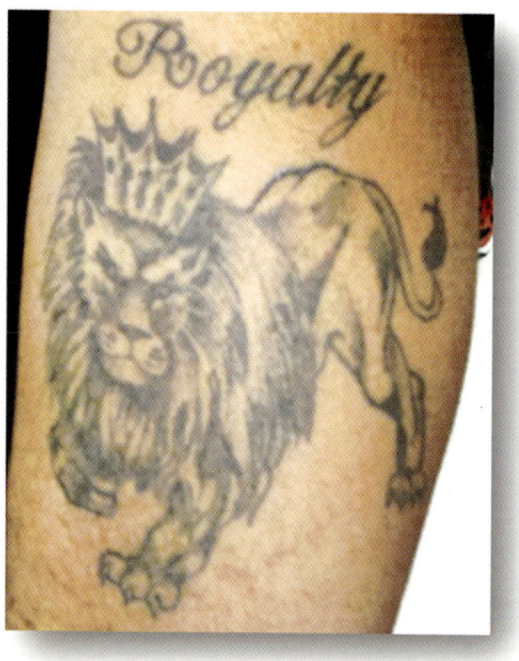

Acknowledgements

I would like to acknowledge the people whose gracious input and assistance contributed to the writing of this book.

- The many family, friends, patients, and acquaintances that donated a photo (and a story) of their body art in an effort to educate and inform the current and next generations.
- My wife Melanie, and three sons, Alex, Nick, and JR, for their unwavering love, support, and sacrifice.
- Sherman Moon, for his ongoing counsel and proofreading.
- Martin Kelly, for his advice, proofreading, and personal account of his first tattoo.
- Maria Shine Stewart for her editing for high school students.
- The Hall family, by blood and marriage, for their unconditional love and support as we try to leave a legacy of pride and unity for future generations.

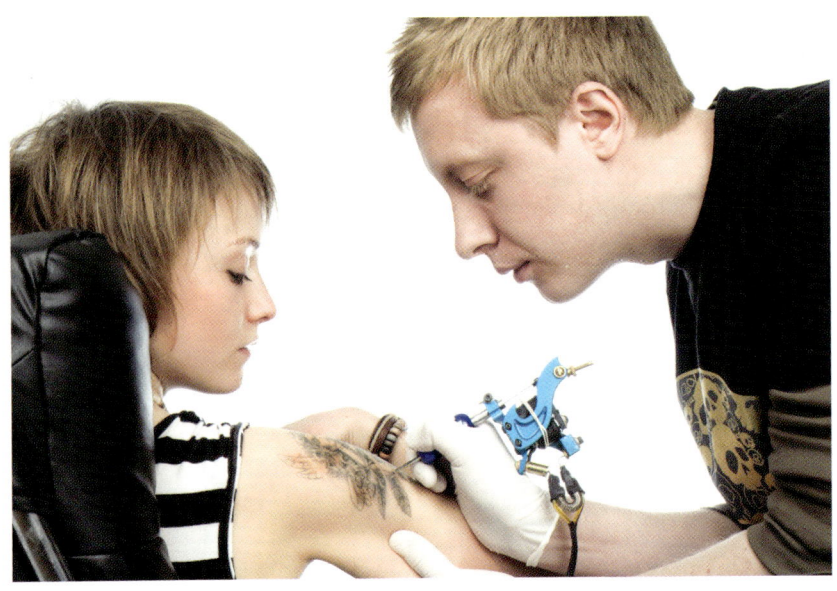

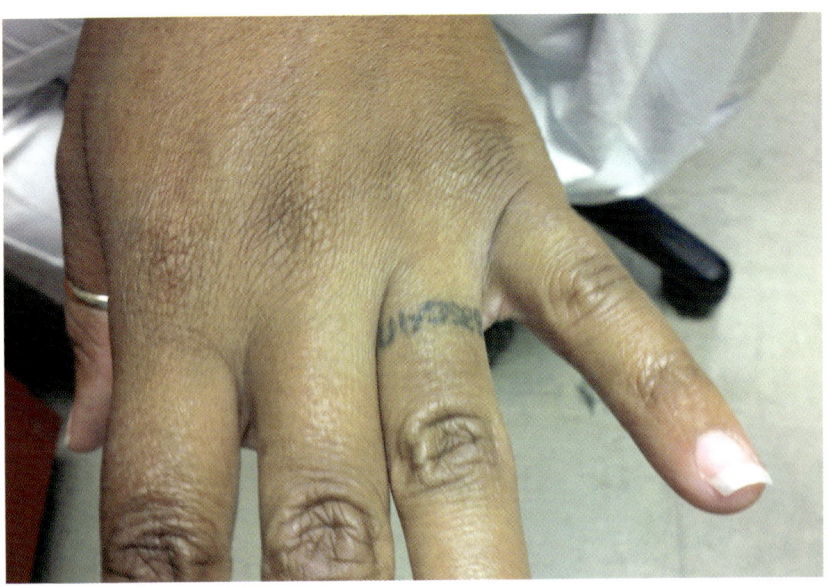

Chapters

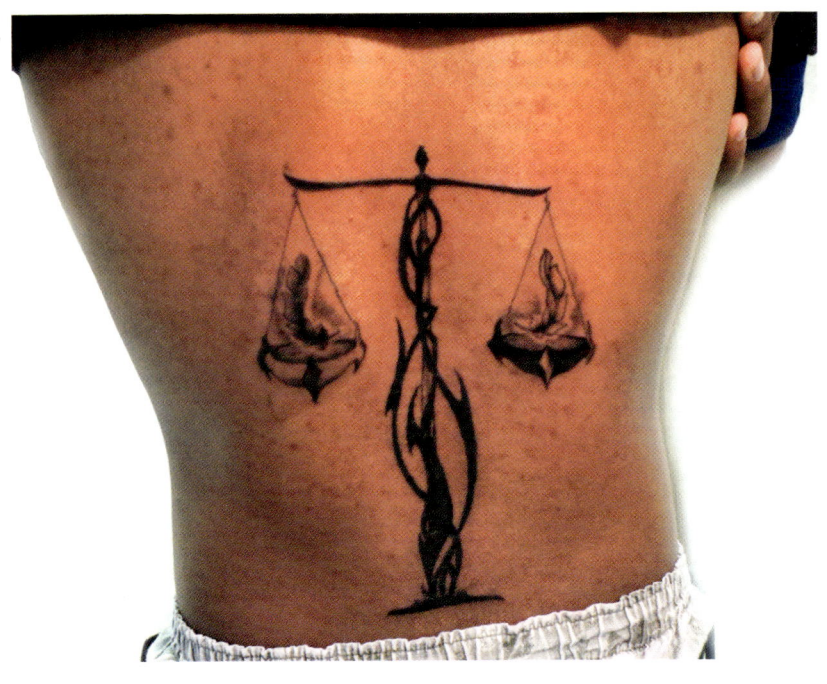

Take a balanced approach to body art.

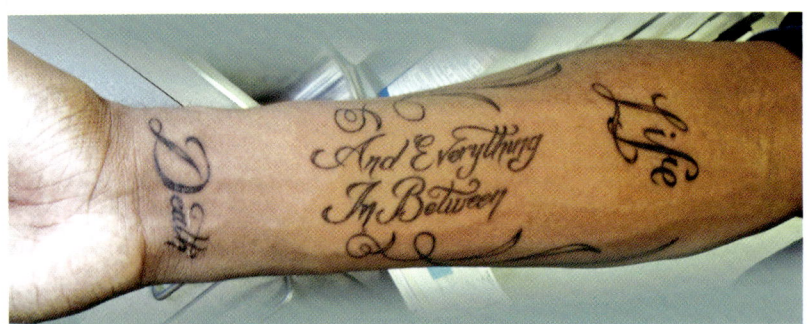

Chapter 1: Trends and Tattoos

While tattoos have been around almost as long as man has walked on two feet, it's important to understand the modern health implications, the social statement some tattoos make, and the natural course (including fading or blurring) of tattoos throughout the rest of your life.

Body art, and the right to get body art, is a personal decision to be made with care and thought. Why? Because tattoos are

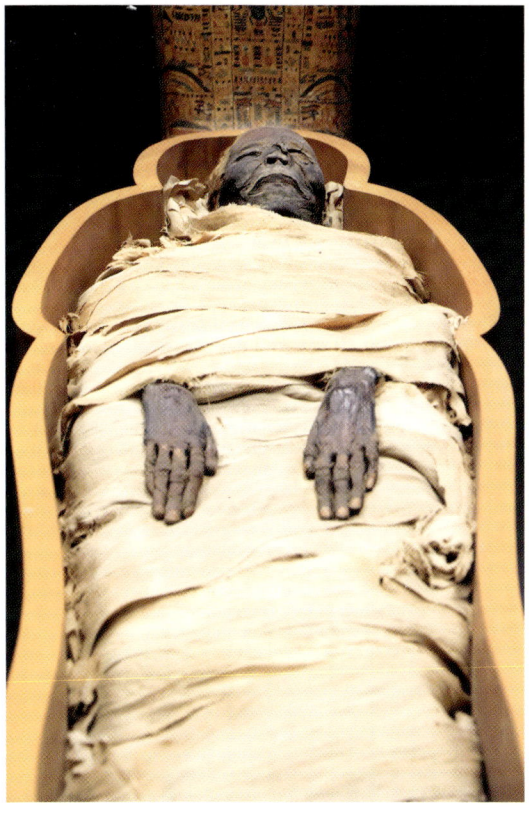

permanent (or at least should be considered permanent) and the final outcome, good or bad, smart or dumb, sexy or not, will be with you the rest of your life. You will be buried with your tattoo. Given the seriousness, and permanence, of the decision, a considerable amount of personal research should go into the process.

The history of human kind is filled with *dermatography* (that means permanent markings on the body.)

Tattoos, as we know them, have been found on mummies (and daddies) and other ancient beings for thousands of years. These permanent markings have been used to identify and track slaves, show military rank, display marital status, and so on. Tattoos have adorned tribal priestesses and labeled escaped prisoners.

In the medical world, tattoos have been used to cover unsightly scars, fill in skin pigment in people with vitiligo (patches of lost skin color), and add normal-appearing pigment after plastic surgery. These thoughtful applications would not be available without the widespread use and

> ### *Tattoo (Tat-too):*
> Tahitian term for "the result of tapping."
> *The act or practice of marking the skin with indelible patterns, pictures, legends, etc., by making punctures in it and inserting pigments.*

experimentation of our tattooed ancestors.

The idea of getting a tattoo is quite common, and for all the people who have taken the plunge and gotten one, there are millions more who are in the learning and thinking phase. Some people estimate that over half the U.S. population between 18 and 50 years has considered getting body art. The percentage of individuals below the poverty level (under age 40) with tattoos probably does exceed 50%, and in some urban areas the percentage is much higher.

Usually, people who consider getting a tattoo -- and then talk themselves out it -- usually do so for understandable reasons.

- They realize that they change their mind too frequently to make a decision that they can't reverse.
- They frequently get bored with hair styles or clothing styles, so a permanent design on their body would be hated in a few months.
- Their future career choices (or employers) make getting an obvious tattoo a bad idea, and they want to keep their career options open.

- They aren't impulsive, and data shows most first tattoos were done on an impulse, on a dare, or with alcohol or drugs involved.
- They don't want to be (wrongfully) "judged" as wild, cheap, and less intelligent than others. (I know it's not fair that people judge others, but some do.)
- They don't like how old tattoos look on older people who have them.

The people that went ahead and got the tattoo are an interesting bunch as well. The early adopters, the ones who have had tattoos all along, were an independent, strong-minded, and decisive bunch. They made a decision and didn't look back. Most never regretted it. This first group of body art fans were the bikers, 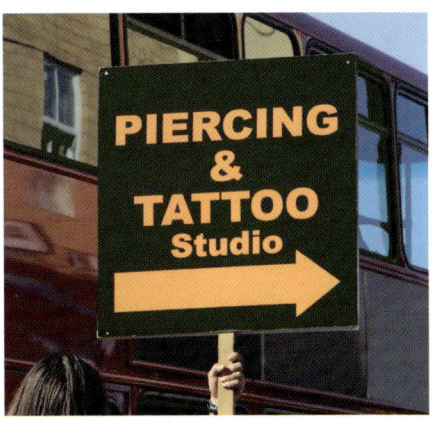 fraternity brothers, soldiers, and prisoners . . . all macho types who were decisive and acted without regret! They were the trend-setters to today's very commonplace tattoo. But back then, the tattoo came with status, membership, or just pure rebellion. The tattoo made a statement, and generally, the person wearing it was proud of the statement they wanted to make.

Other people admired the rebellion or strength of conviction required to get a tattoo and thought: "I want to be strong, and self-assured like them." So others, slowly "got the nerve" to get inked. Sailors, admiring the strength of their captains (and their colorful forearm with a sinking ship), would show their rite of passage by getting a tattoo. Some fraternities (both college and lodge brothers) across the country began to demand a small tattoo as a sign of brotherhood and loyalty.

In the western world, until the late 20th century, the tattoo was almost exclusively a "man thing," and only a "manly woman" would even think of getting one. With the 1960's, the rebellion of youths against "the Establishment" -- or the conservative authoritarian system of those in charge -- brought a wave of opposites. If conformity said one thing, the youths in the sixties HAD to do the opposite. Men began growing long hair while women would crop their hair short. Sex, which had been saved for after marriage, became "free" and non-committed. And tattoos, which stayed among only the macho men in the past, became a sign of a woman's independent spirit as well in some circles.

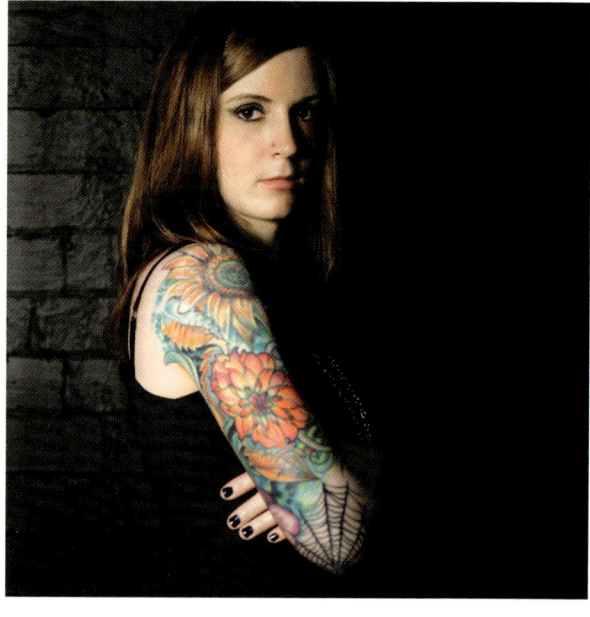

In the west, women's adoption of tattoos started small and slowly grew over time. Like a pendulum swinging, American women have recently passed men in the number who are getting tattoos, and the small flower or bird that women used to get is being displaced with larger more elaborate designs that cover much more of the body. By contrast, in the Orient, where tattooing still remains a fine art with centuries of history and tradition, women have always been the main people with this type of decoration, and they enjoy widespread acceptance.

What do I need to know about getting a tattoo?

When you have a big decision to make, like getting a tattoo, you should remember that it may affect the rest of your life. In addition to the usual tattoo questions, like "What design should I get?" and "Where should it go?". . .are some even more important questions that you should get answered:

- *What are the possible side effects of tattoos?*
- *What health risks exist, and how real are they?*
- *What am I giving up by getting a tattoo?*
- *How hard is it to remove if I don't like it?*

This book was not written to persuade you not to get a tattoo. Instead, it gives you all the information you need to make a thoughtful and educated decision with both your head and your heart.

The fact is: A lot of famous and popular people have tattoos, and, as a culture, some of us like to copy them in dress, talk, and action. Almost universally, fashion and trends are set by famous and prominent people. But these same famous people have trouble with permanent decisions as well. Angelina Jolie had her first husband's name "Billy Bob" tattooed on her upper arm. When they broke up, the name had to be removed. The actress Megan Fox is

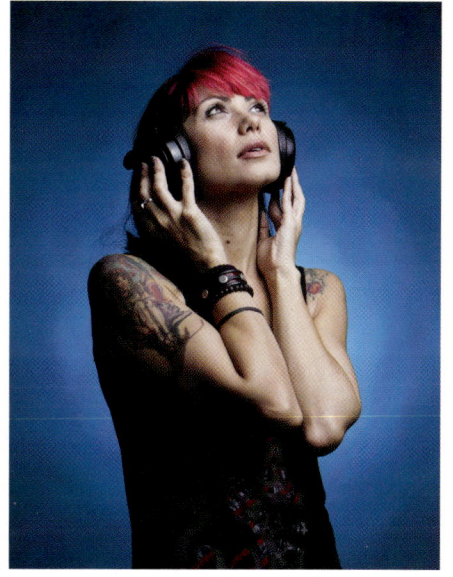

getting her tattoos removed because she would spend too much time covering them when they interfered with roles she wanted to play or an image she wanted to project. Actors in Hollywood are also getting their tattoos removed because now the bold and unique trend is to be tattoo-free. Yes, this "permanent" trend is now fading in some circles.

Trends (or fads) are social habits that start with one person and then, as people copy the habit or fashion, it spreads across the community (and sometimes the nation). Some trends last for many years (women's high-heeled shoes, for example), while other trends are more fleeting (such as gold teeth). A popular movie has an actress with long curly hair, and hair salons across the country show an increase in that particular style for a while. A year later, the same actress can be replaced by a more popular (and usually younger) actress in the spotlight who wears short hair; then, short styles will become popular. This example is useful for at least two reasons as you consider getting a tattoo:

1. *Styles come and go. . .* How are you going to choose a tattoo that will stay in style the rest of your life?
2. *If you are the type that likes to be "in style" (the latest fashions and newest electronics, for example),* in five years, how are you going to explain – to others or to yourself -- a tattoo that has gone out of style?

In a Pew Research survey of people age 50 and over, the majority of the respondents felt the increased number of tattoos

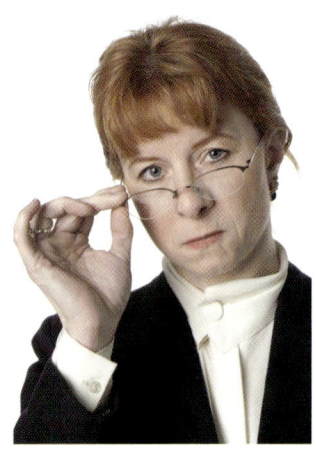

was a change for the worse. In the adult groups younger than 50, the majority felt tattoos had no effect on society, but 22 to 32% still felt the change was for the worse. Overall, 40% of people felt tattoos were not a positive influence on society. When getting a tattoo, the 4 out of 10 that have a negative view of tattoos have to be considered if you intend to apply for a job, look for a promotion, hope for admission to a special college or program, or pick a life partner. You will be carrying a visible mark that some others view unfavorably, no matter your reason for getting the tattoo.

> ➤ *Consider this: 1 out of 20 people with a tattoo will attempt to cover it with another tattoo!*

Imagine trying to choose a tattoo that can also be covered successfully by another, more trendy one. You can't, and why would you? People's needs to remove, alter, or re-do tattoos have built a huge industry of tattoo removal by laser, cream, acid, surgery, and so on. Chemists are developing a tattoo ink that is more easily "removable," but only time will tell if it will be safe and effective.

Change, and changing times, means changing culture. In the sixties and seventies, no one wore athletic shoes unless they were in a school gym. Now, people wear athletic shoes to formal events. In the 1970's, bell bottom pants were everywhere. Now, you would be a laughing stock wearing them in most settings.

Women's skirts, and for that matter, men's shorts, rise and fall with the changing trends. One year mini-skirts are "in" and the next they are "out." The following year, long shorts go past the knee, and the next – they are even lower. Look at basketball shorts! What if men still had the short-shorts of the 1980's? Men

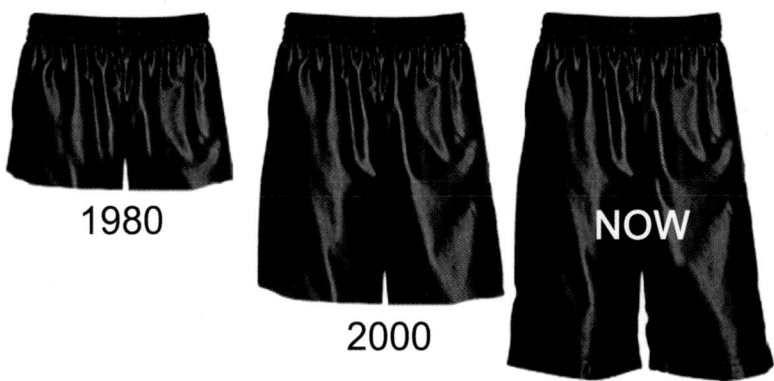

1980

2000

NOW

felt completely normal in very short pants back then, but now we smile at how "stupid" that fashion looked. How can you choose a permanent decoration for your body that will <u>not</u> go out of style? That is a thorny question. It is impossible to make time – or styles – stand still. No one can predict what will be the hot trend of the future.

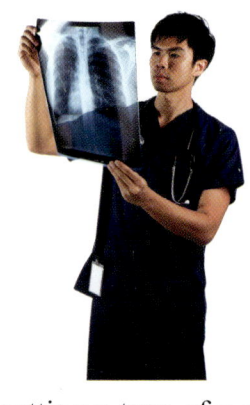

Not only is finding a "timeless" tattoo design a problem, you are also limited in your choice of colors. Each color complicates the process and increases the risk for allergic reaction, infection, and final outcome. The ink colors available are growing by the day as different mixtures are developed. The most vivid colors traditionally contained what is called "heavy metals." These made the tattoo darker and deeper, but they also made getting a type of x-ray called an MRI more complicated. If you got a medical condition that required repeated MRI's as a way to track the disease, and your heavy metal tattoo disrupts the images (and begins to burn), the decision to get a tattoo could literally affect your life and health!

And what about your calling or work in life? You may not be sure just yet. But suppose you decide to become a minister or deacon at church, and you just happen to also have a tattoo. Just read Leviticus 19:28: "Ye shall not make any cuttings in your flesh for the dead,

> 26 ¶ Ye shall not eat *any thing* with the blood: neither shall ye use enchantment, nor observe times.
> 27 Ye shall not round the corners of your heads, neither shalt thou mar the corners of thy beard.
> 28 Ye shall not make any cuttings in your flesh for the dead, nor print any marks upon you: I *am* the LORD.
>
> LEVITICUS 20
> he shall surely be put to de the people of the land stone him with stones.
> 3 And I will set my against that man, and wi him off from among his ple; because he hath giv his seed unto Molech, to my sanctuary, and to pr my holy name.
> 4 And if the people land do any way hide

nor *print any marks on you*: I am the LORD." More progressive churches probably won't mind the tattoo, but other more stringent institutions might.

If you know the health risks, the social implications, the changing trends, the possible employment ramifications, and still decide to get a tattoo, that's great! Your eyes and ears are open to reality. You will have made an informed decision, and you will most likely be happy with the outcome, and be at peace with your decision the rest of your life.

However, if you impulsively dive into getting one on a dare, or after a drink, or while mourning a death, or while madly in love, you will most likely live to regret it.

Because there are also some unexpected health consequences possible when getting a tattoo, please know all the risks and all the facts before making this very important decision.

The health and social ramifications of getting a tattoo are many, and the wise consumer will thoughtfully and carefully consider each aspect ranging from:

- infection,
- to scarring,
- to changing trends.

Read this book cover to cover. It was purposely made to read in one or two sittings. Consider its information, and remember that it is not designed to talk you out of getting a tattoo. Above all, it is designed to give you all of the information you need to make a decision with which you can live.

Your life will absolutely include regrets sooner or later: Everyone has them. This book is designed to make getting a tattoo or piercing <u>not</u> one of your regrets.

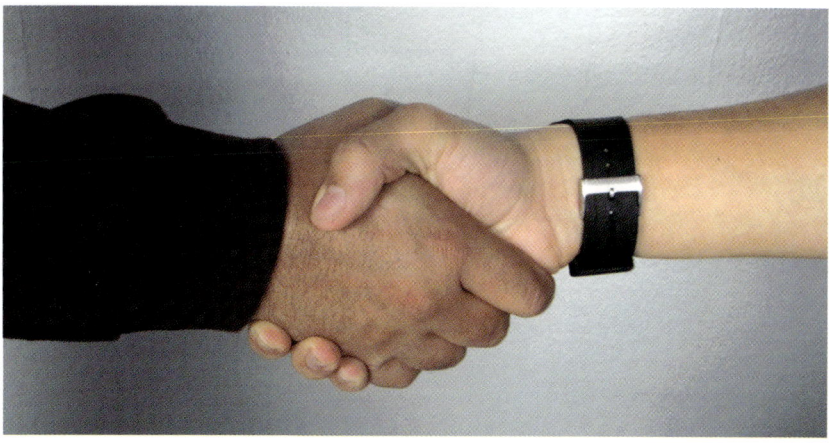

Chapter 2: How a Tattoo Is Done

Permanent body art, in the form of what we now call tattoos, has been a part of human tradition since the dawn of time. Egyptian mummies have been discovered not only wrapped, but also tattooed. For whatever reason -- religious, tribal, or occupation -- there has always been a fraction of society who

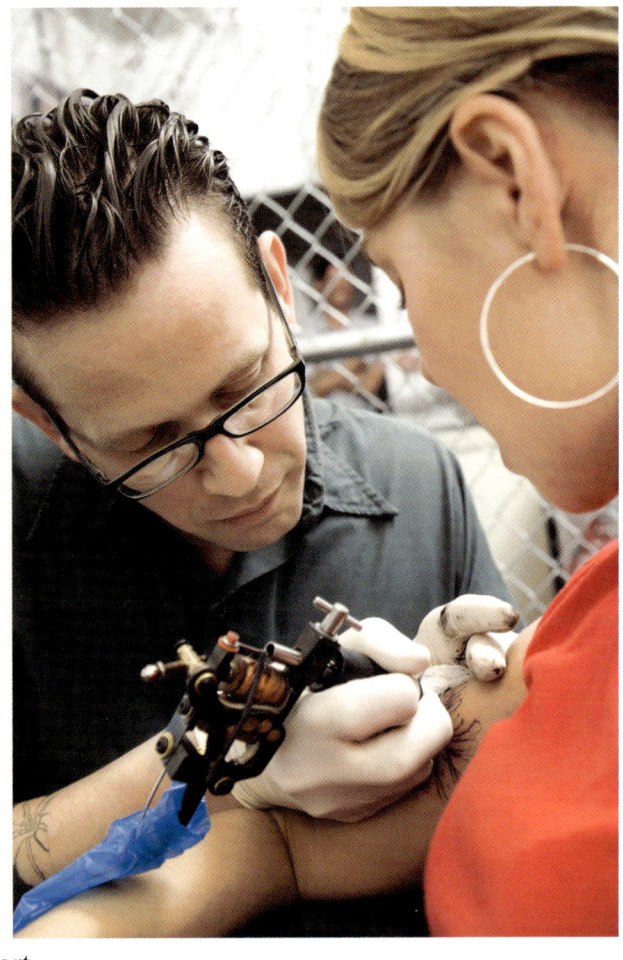

sought out body art.

For the majority of western civilization, the tradition had been reserved for men, and not just any men, but ones with rugged backgrounds and traditions. Sailors, soldiers, and outlaws were all renowned for "sporting" their tattoos.

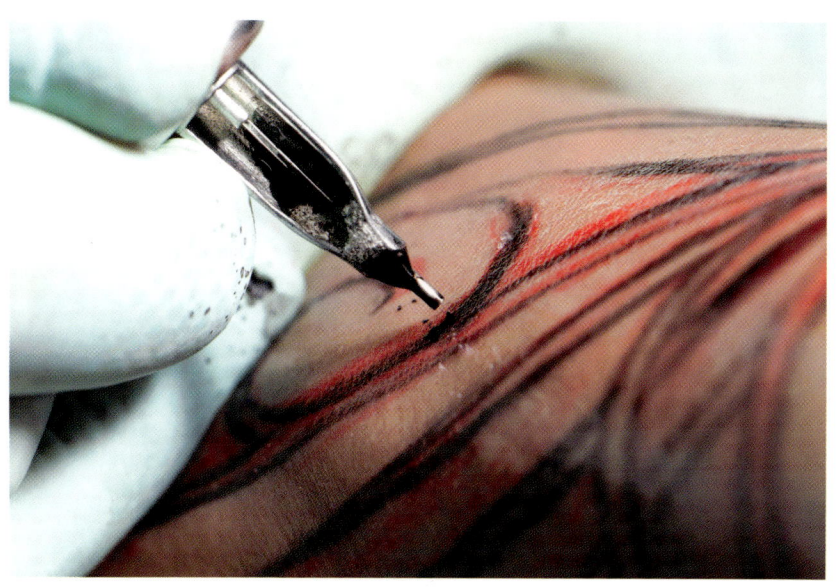

While the men who got tattoos were rough, the process of getting a tattoo was manly and grueling as well. The tattoo artist (who frequently was NOT an artist at all) would use a piece of sharp metal, dip it into whatever they used for ink (soot, dirt, rust, etc.) and pierce the top layer of skin, leaving behind the dot of ink. Each dot formed the basis for the final picture. Like the pixels (colored dots) on a computer screen, the art was "drawn" one point/stick at a time. The entire process was slow, painful, and frequently left an image that was crude. Using modern machinery, and developed technique, the modern tattooist can be an artist extraordinaire! Using the body as a canvas, with inks, dilutions, mixtures, and skill, the artist can literally paint a landscape on your body.

While the tattooing process is age-old, as technology has advanced, sophisticated machinery has replaced the crude single needle with ink. More knowledge of the potential for infection has led to safer practices. Disposable needles, safer ink mixtures, and inspections by local health departments have significantly decreased the risk and

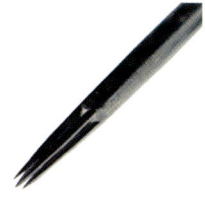

occurrence of infections related to the tattooing process when done at a professional and healthy location.

The needles have grown more sophisticated as well, and come in a variety of shapes and bundles so that larger areas (than a single dot) can be done much more quickly. While a tattoo on the open sea in the 1800's may have taken months to complete, modern tattoos, even somewhat complicated ones, can be done in a single visit.

How is a Tattoo Done?

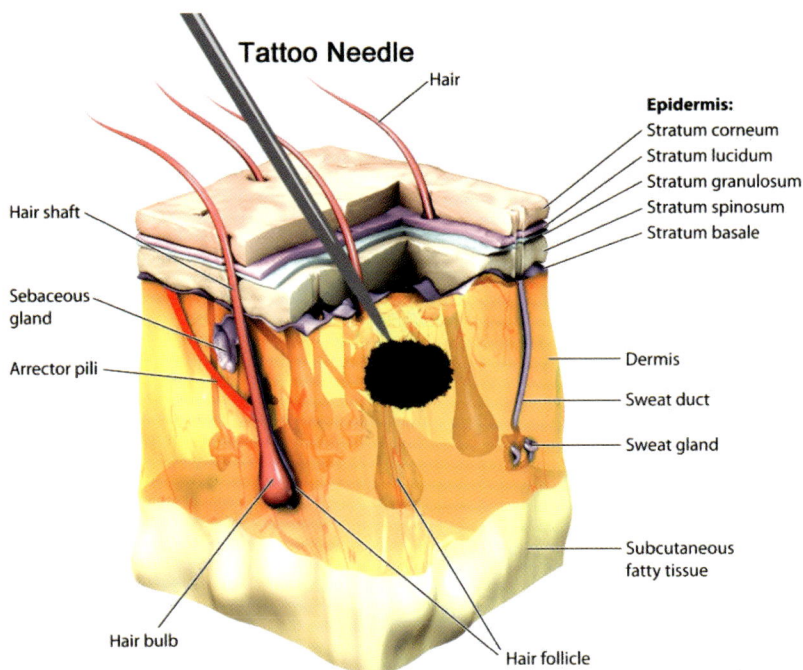

The tattoo needle must go through several layers of skin before reaching the dermis.
Any virus, bacteria, dirt, or other substance on the surface of the skin will be pushed into the body.

Simply put, your skin has six layers, the first five layers (which make up the epidermis) change and renew with time, and the under-layer (or dermis) which never changes. In the normal body, the epidermis protects the dermis from injury, scarring, and staining. The body can then get tanned, coated, painted, and so on, without permanently changing or impacting the dermis. A change in the dermis, otherwise known as a permanent scar, is usually to be avoided. Tattooing bypasses the protection provided by the epidermal layers, and allows a permanent design to be embedded in a layer that cannot be removed by the body. Understand the permanence, and try to imagine how you might feel about that should your taste in body art change in the future.

During the actual tattooing process, the ink is injected in little pin-points by one ink dot per stick. In the distant past, designs would take weeks to complete. Now, with the aid of electricity and modern technology, the tattoo needles are sophisticated, and one may stick 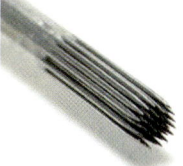 the dermis multiple times a second. Needle bundles can do larger areas at one time. Despite the change in the speed of the process (elaborate designs can be done in a fraction of the time it took years ago), it is still just a stick and a tiny drop of ink that are the basis of tattooing.

The tattoo artist uses a tattoo gun similar to the one shown here. The ink is now vacuum-drawn into the ink gun and rapidly 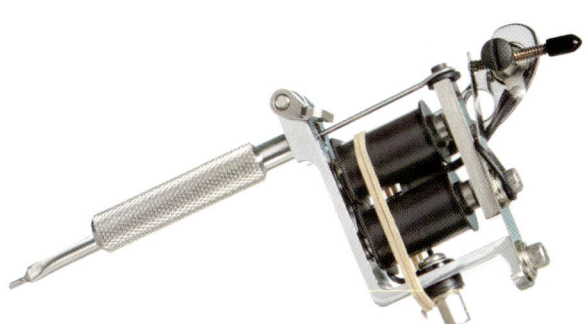 injected into the lower level of the skin, where it will permanently remain.

The tattoo artist will first clean the area thoroughly, killing all bacteria and viruses, and then apply a layer of petroleum jelly to help control dye contamination of adjacent areas. The ink is then 'injected" immediately under the skin. The design, one color at a time, is then drawn and filled in. The dye may ooze out of the tattoo during some of the healing process. Extreme care should be taken to avoid sun exposure or injury to the skin during the healing process.

Biological "reactions" occur during the tattooing healing process that help to preserve the tattoo, and there are other reactions that could ruin it entirely. Naturally, when a foreign substance is introduced into it, the body reacts by first isolating the substance, and then removing it, if it can. The initial inflammatory response brings fluid to the site (swelling), increases the blood supply (redness), and causes tenderness and pain (to avoid further injury). These functional body responses, and time, are all necessary for natural healing. Normally, they keep our bodies on track.

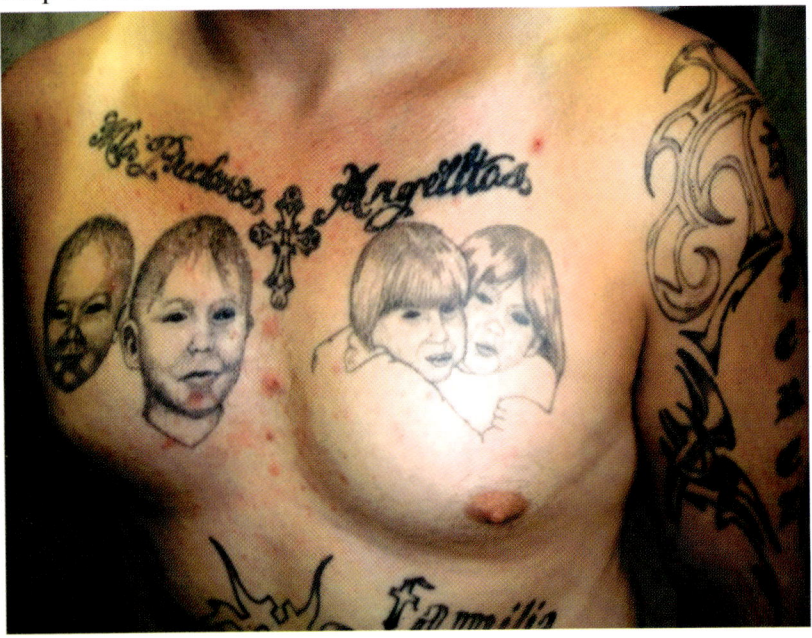

If too much of an inflammatory response occurs, however, an infection can result, the design can be negatively affected, or the dye color can be changed or transformed to something not expected. Occasionally the inflammation will even compromise the body's immune status, and an outbreak of shingles, psoriasis, herpes, or something else can be "allowed" to re-activate. These are serious consequences that cannot be predicted in advance.

Do people get "addicted" to tattoos and piercing?

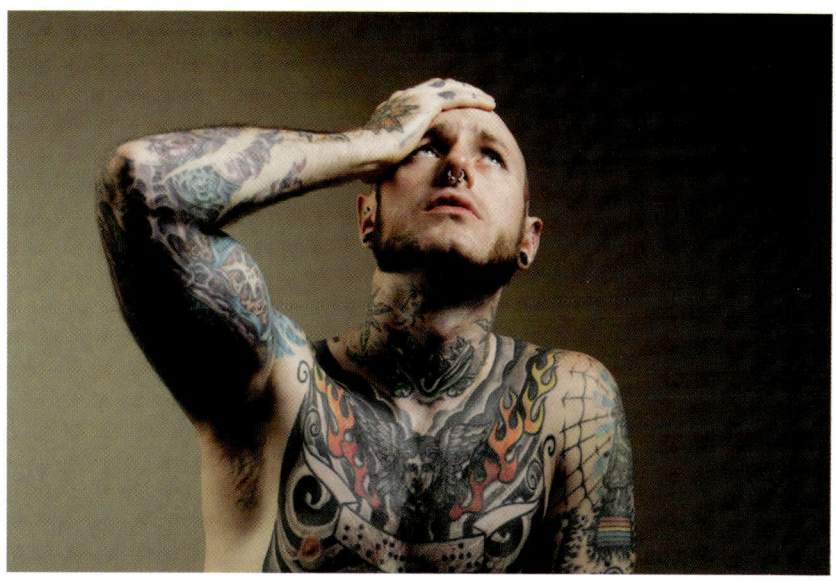

Some people confess that the actual process of getting a tattoo is pleasurable to them. To these people, like acupuncture, the needle sticks are paradoxically "fun, therapeutic, or exciting." This curious phenomenon may be explained by the release of endorphins and other pleasurable substances in response to the stimulating effect of the needle sticks. Endorphins naturally occur in the brain and are responsible for feeling good. Exercising also releases endorphins. Many of the individuals who ultimately get addicted to tattoos are usually the same ones who have addiction problems with other substances. To them, the process is still painful, but like piercing and acupuncture, can sometimes have an interestingly pleasurable effect. The piercing of the skin causes pain that is mediated by numerous nerve endings under the skin. These nerves also begin biochemical reactions which lead to the release of multiple substances related to healing. These chemicals have some properties that give a pleasurable sensation to some people, while others just feel pain. Occasionally, those that get "aroused" by pain, and the body's consequences of painful stimulation, seek to repeat the process. They are not so much doing it for the tattoo or piercing outcome as they are the process of getting body art. These individuals "run out" of spots to put their new tattoo or piercing ideas. Some of these individuals bask in the attention and "fearless daring" that is required for whole body tattoos and multiple piercings. Others may regret these compulsions later in life.

How can you tell if you will enjoy tattoo or piercing? If you

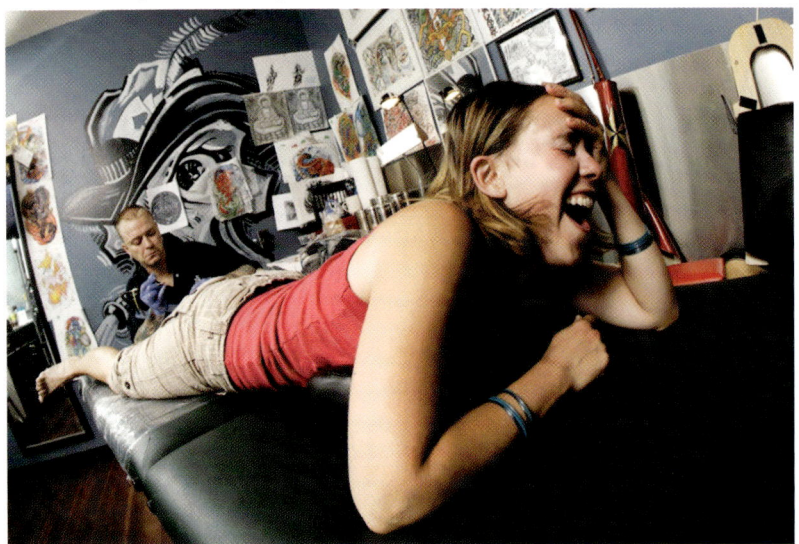

are the type that takes medication for pain, rather than just tolerating it without help, you will likely not get "addicted" to the

pain aspect of the tattoo or piercing process.

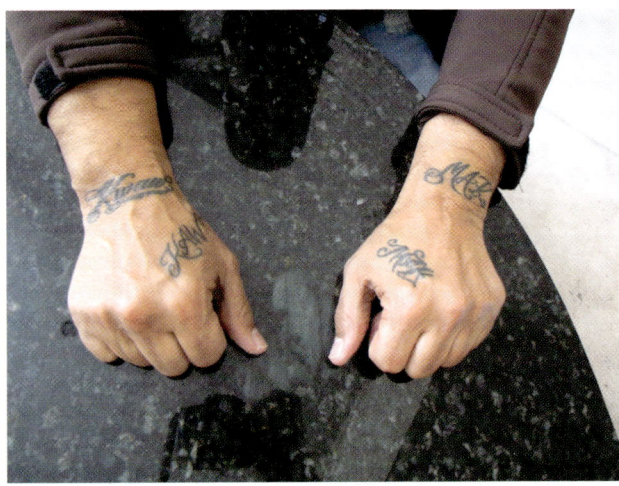

Chapter 3: The Ink

There are various issues surrounding the inks used in the tattoo process. Some artists feel the true value and rarity of their designs lay in their special ink mixtures and 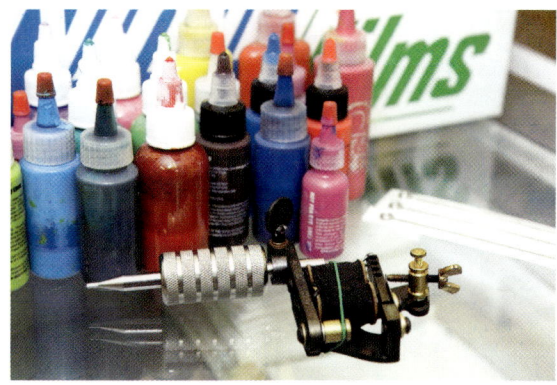 compounds. These inks give the tattoo its quality and vividness. Some inks give a lasting deep rich color, others react poorly with the sun, while others fade somewhat with time regardless of sun exposure. Choosing the right ink for you will also take some research. Take time to do it. The ingredients in the ink vary by manufacturer and each component carries a possibility of an allergic reaction, in addition to the health unknowns associated with having these sometimes toxic substances placed in the body. Sample ingredients include:

BLACK: iron oxides, or carbon

BLUE: copper salts, sodium aluminum silicate, calcium

BROWN: iron oxides

GREEN: chromium oxide, Malachite, Ferrocyanides, Lead chromate, Monoazo pigment.

ORANGE: disazodiarylide, disazopyrazolone, or cadmium seleno-sulfide.

RED: Iron oxide, cinnabar, cadmium red, iron oxide, or napthol.

YELLOW: Iron oxide, cadmium yellow, ochres, curcuma yellow, chrome yellow, or disazodiarylide.

VIOLET: manganese ammonium pyrophosphate, quinacridone, dioxazine/carbazole, and aluminum salts.

WHITE: lead carbonate, titanium dioxide, barium sulfate, or zinc oxide.

A quick review of the inks reveals a host of metals and metal-mixtures, which also explains the problems with x-ray machines. Metals can interfere with scans at times. Potential issues with new airport screening devices should also be considered. As mentioned, depending on the ink mixture, some individuals are warned against having Magnetic Resonance Imaging given the degree of metals left under the skin. With high levels of iron oxide, there is the potential for burns or distortions of the tattoo caused by the MRI process. An MRI can be a very important, even life-saving, tool to diagnose illness or injury. Know your risks of losing access to this critical invention.

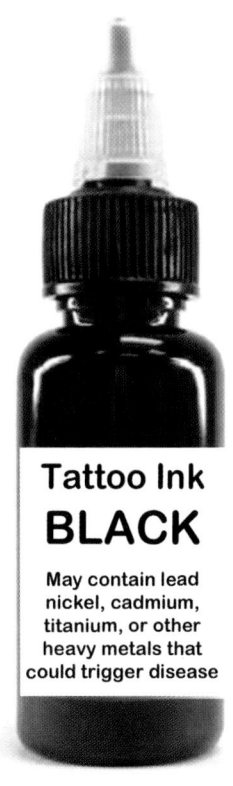

Tattoo Ink
BLACK
May contain lead nickel, cadmium, titanium, or other heavy metals that could trigger disease

A medical journal published a report of a younger gentleman getting an MRI and during the exam he reported an intense burning of certain parts of the tattoo on his arm and shoulder. The pain continued so he returned the next day to the emergency room for further treatment. The black ink contained enough metal that the machine (which uses a very large magnet) began to move the ink under his skin. This is shocking, and true.

The ink manufacturer confirmed that iron oxide in the ink was the most likely culprit.

Another report published in an OB/GYN journal showed another case of a woman with a lower back tattoo that "burned" during the procedure but fortunately showed no greater or obvious reaction.

Despite these issues, tattoos are generally not a problem when having an MRI procedure. A really deeply

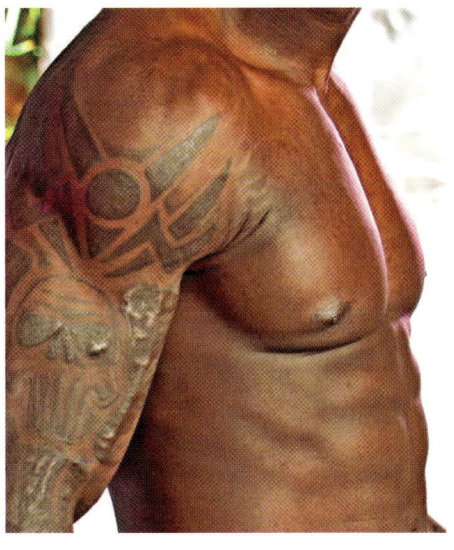

colored tattoo, however, made with iron oxide should put the possibility of a reaction in your head. So consider: What is more important to you? An image on your body that suggests a free spirit – or the freedom to have your body scanned without worry, should the need arise?

Ink Rejection?

The body has a natural ability to renew and clean itself. It will commonly reject or attempt to remove the pigment as a foreign body: this is a natural and functional reaction. Are you surprised? People will see this process when the tattoo takes longer to heal than expected, or some parts of the tattoo (commonly the red part) takes longer to heal than the other parts of the design.

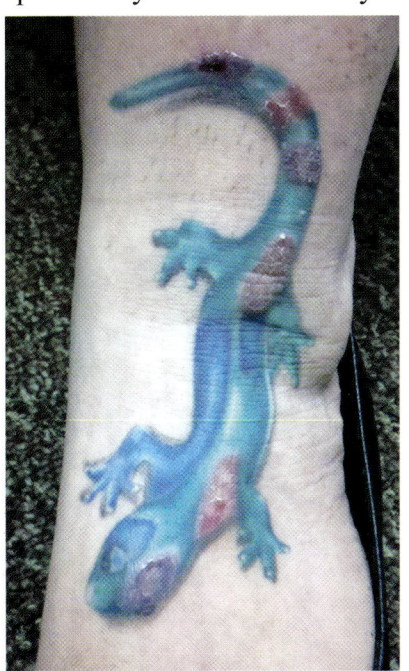

Notice the RED dye reaction while the blue & green are okay

Some colors are notorious – or known for -- causing an allergic reaction while others are less offensive. Reds cause the most allergic reactions across the board due to their unique components. If you have a lot of allergies, you will want to

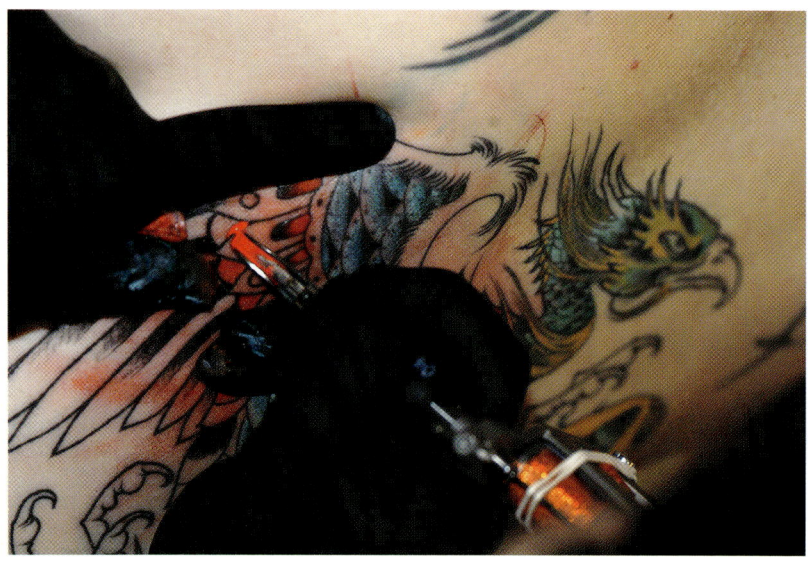

investigate the ink components and review your particular allergies (example: napthol) before you get a fancy tattoo that goes wild during the healing process.

With all of these metal and chemical ingredients, the majority of the common inks are "toxic" in one way or another. Toxic, for our purposes, means that exposure to the human body, in an adequate amount, can cause sickness (cancer, organ failure, etc.), or even death. Small amounts of ink may be tolerated very well in some individuals. Yet in others, it may, after 20 years, cause a medical problem. In the same way that some smokers get lung cancer (after 30 years) and others never do, the inks with toxic heavy metals may affect some individuals and not others. Because such substances are used in tiny amounts, and in the dermis of the skin, most people have no problem from them. But be aware that the risk is there, and it is a real one.

Another new consideration is a recently released "easier to remove" tattoo ink. Infinite ink is a tattooing ink that apparently lasts as long as conventional tattoos, yet is easier to remove if you decide you don't like your body art anymore. Tattoo removal procedures have improved over time, but it's still costly and painful, but use of a "removable ink" might give a less painful option if you tend to change your mind frequently.

Currently there is little FDA oversight of the inks and the compounds used to make them. Most inks use commercial substances commonly used to color ceramics or paints, and certainly were not developed for application in people.

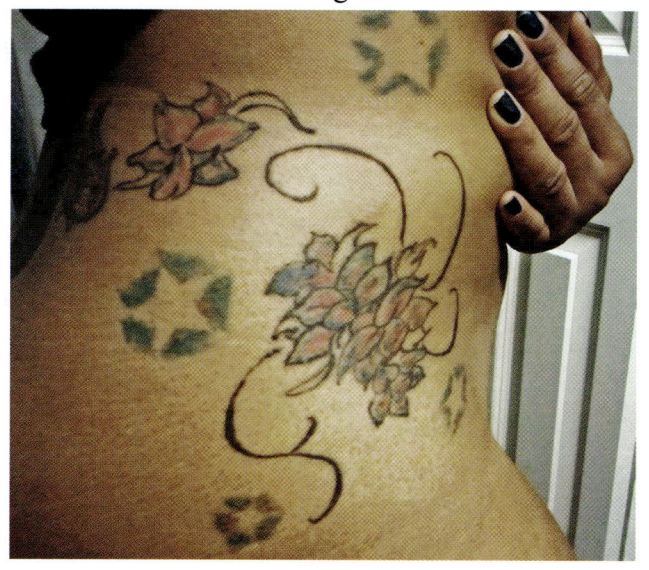

As news has spread on these industrial products used in biological applications, the Go Green movement began to really encourage organic products in their dyes which are safer, healthier, and provide more peace of mind.

All inks aren't ready to go when they arrive at the tattoo studio. The ink itself may come to the dealer as a powder or a concentrate that needs to be diluted. What substance they use to dilute or dissolve the ink is also critically important. A number of outbreaks of water borne infections have sprung up when tattooists used tap water to dissolve the ink. If water is used, always insist upon "sterile" or "distilled" water. It is your body. Other liquids used to dilute the ink include ethyl alcohol, witch hazel, propylene glycol, glycerin, or even Listerine! Time will tell which substances are safest and most effective.

Remember: Inks can get contaminated when opened.
- Whatever the technician puts the ink in <u>should be sterile</u>.
- Whatever is mixed with ink <u>should be sterile</u>.
- Whatever tubing the ink flows through <u>should be sterile</u>.
- You should <u>know everything</u> that's in the ink.
- Because many inks were not developed for this purpose, there is no telling how sterile or unsterile the powder was prior to delivery to the shop.

All of these ink questions need to be asked and answered. Speak up for yourself!

A new "Go Green" movement is rapidly growing in the tattoo world where only naturally occurring inks are used. These non-metal inks will undoubtedly improve the health outcomes for people down the road, so always ask about <u>a natural source</u> for inks. If you do have a natural ink source, the risk for allergic rejection should be much less.

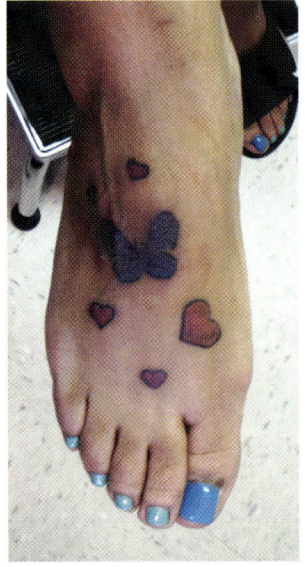

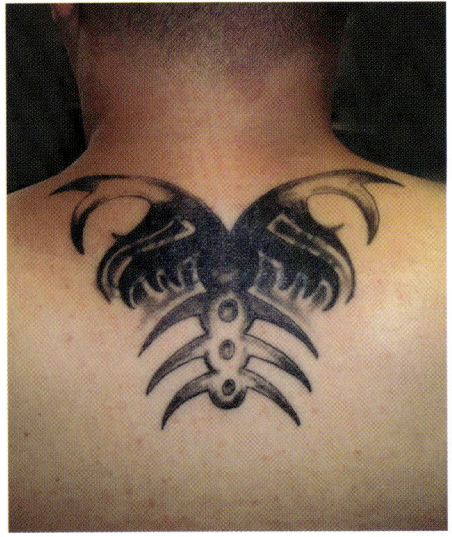

Chapter 4: What could go wrong?

One of the problems with sticking yourself a thousand times a minute and injecting, hopefully noninfectious, ink into your skin, is that not everyone has the outcome they expect. In your mind, you may imagine a wonderful result with no problems. In your body, however, infections with hepatitis, a type of liver infection, antibiotic resistant bacteria, or even HIV/AIDS are a

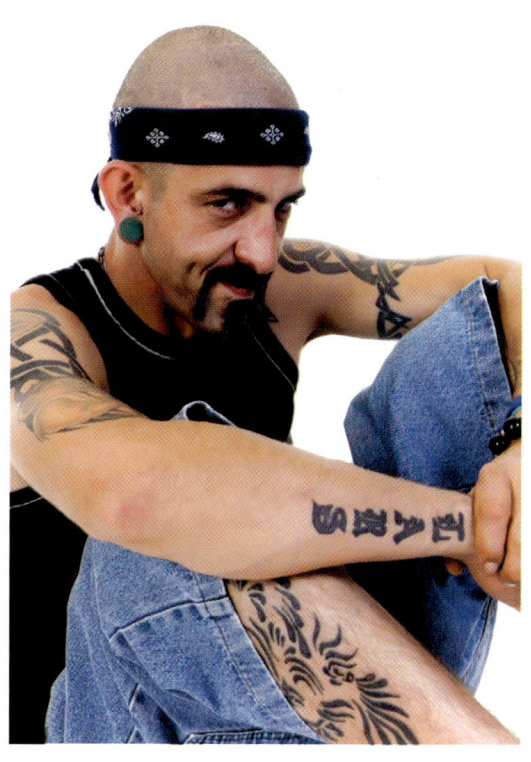

possibility with each tattoo visit, in fact with each needle stick!

The recent increasing popularity of dermagraphic art (tattoos) and body piercing has caused states and local health departments to begin to track clusters of infections, especially Staph infections (MRSA) and hepatitis. Every time the skin is broken, bacteria from the needle, the tattooist, or the surface of the skin of the person can be injected into the blood. Once the bacteria or virus is in the blood it can duplicate, grow, and possibly infect. Because the needles used are not hollow, like those used to draw blood or give medication, the risk for transmitting any infection is less with tattoo needles. But the risk is still there, and is very real. Health departments across the country see a variety of infections related to tattoos, and by far the most dangerous risk comes from non-licensed tattooists. Those tattoos obtained in prisons, in detention facilities, at halfway houses, or at parties present the greatest risk because people in those places don't have access to proper sterilizing equipment, they haven't been trained on how to prevent infection, and they are poor hand washers!

It is fascinating that many people with tattoos still frown and squirm when they have blood drawn during a doctor's visit (and that is usually only ONE stick), yet they will return time and time again for the repeated sticks of a tattoo without hesitation.

While individual states monitor and inspect tattoo parlors, they simply don't have the resources to provide the oversight needed to prevent infections entirely. There is no guarantee. The same way the health department inspects and advises restaurants to help insure clean practices are being used, they also have the responsibility to control the rate of spreading infections. But they cannot be everywhere at all times.

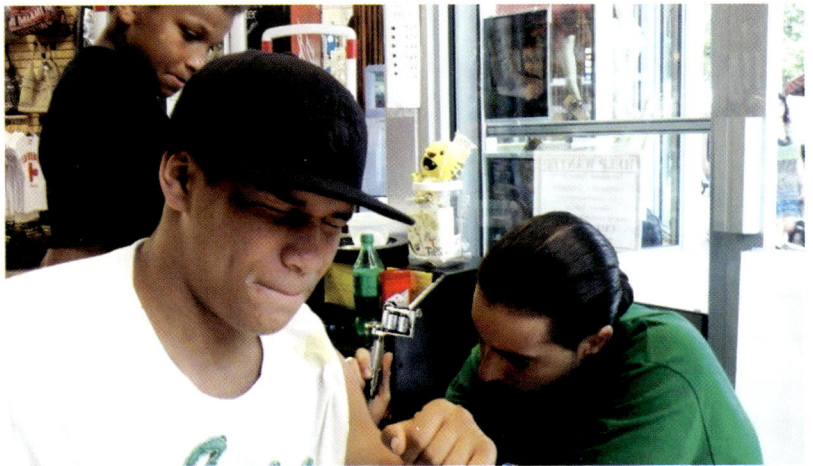

In addition, illegal "private" tattoo artists that organize and attend tattoo parties in homes across the country are a major health threat. There is NO regulation or oversight of these criminals who use poorly cleaned needles and inferior or expired ink. The fact that most who attend have been drinking, coupled with the peer pressure, leads to poor outcomes. <u>No one should entice under-aged teenagers to get a tattoo and a possible life-threatening infection.</u> Scientists are monitoring the incidence of hepatitis as the number of tattoos increase, and some believe that there is a direct relationship in both of these growing numbers.

There are, of course, no definitive or exact answers to how many infections come from getting a tattoo, or even your specific infection rate from each parlor visit. But everyone agrees your chances for acquiring an infection are significantly increased by getting a tattoo. A scientific study published in the journal *Medicine* (Haley RW, Fischer RP, *Commercial tattooing as a potential source of hepatitis C infection, Medicine,* March 2000;80:134-151) showed an increased rate of Hepatitis C in patients who used commercially approved tattoo parlors.

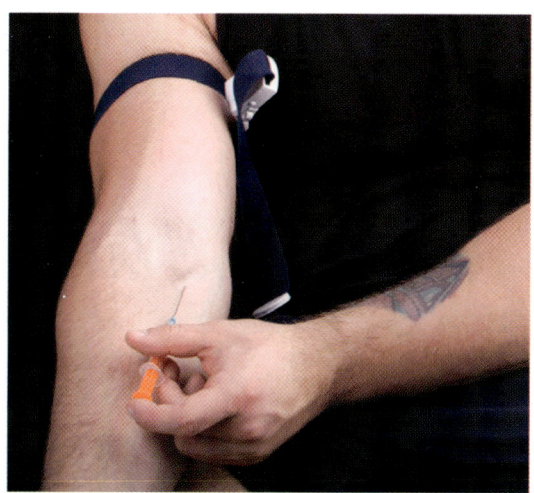

In fact, the researchers found that getting a tattoo from a tattoo parlor gave participants a higher risk of getting Hepatitis C than IV drug use, sexual promiscuity, blood transfusions, or any other measure studied.

The research paper looked at people who already had Hepatitis C and studied how they may have contracted the disease that kills thousands every year. While most would think using intravenous drugs or being sexually promiscuous would increase one's chances of getting Hepatitis C far more than a legally acquired tattoo, it turned out that in this study, a tattoo is far more dangerous, and deadly! Remember that this is just one study and these specific results have not been found elsewhere. If you are going to get a tattoo, a tattoo parlor is by far the best place to go.

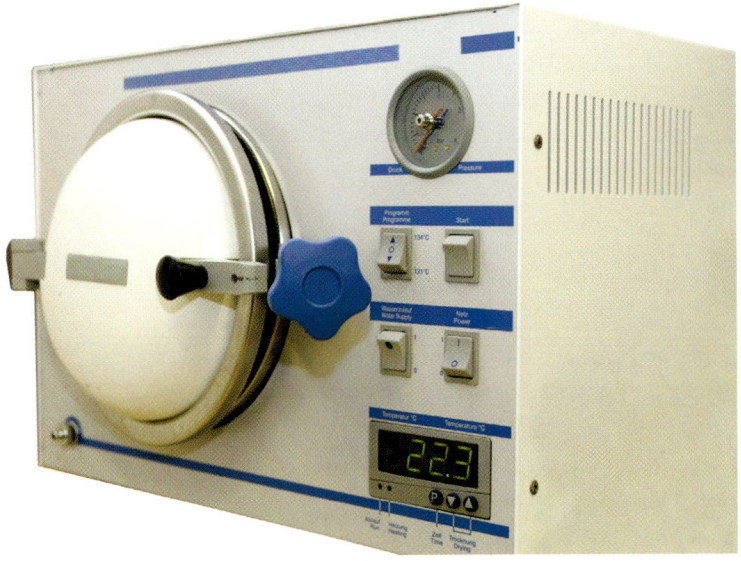

Autoclave Oven

One of the many reasons to use professionals when getting body art is that they use a specialized disinfecting oven designed to kill all bacteria and viruses on their tattooing and piercing equipment. In short, an autoclave is a type of oven that combines:

- **heat (250 degrees Fahrenheit)**
- **steam** at extreme temperatures
- **high pressure**
- **and the absence of air**

in an effort to kill ALL of the bacteria and viruses on a surgical instrument. This prevents the transmission of infections (hepatitis, HIV, staph, strep, and others) as well as promotes proper healing without scarring. All medical professionals (and tattoo/piercing shops) use autoclaves to sterilize their instruments (especially needles).

Autoclaves kill bacteria and viruses that alcohol, bleach, and ammonia cannot. After the instruments come out of the autoclave, they are quickly wrapped to keep sterile for future use. If your body art specialist doesn't have an autoclave, stay away from their equipment!

Did I get Hepatitis C from this tattoo?

Other studies have confirmed that when there is an increase in tattooed people, there is also an increased incidence of Hepatitis C. The National Institute of Health has not issued a position or recommendation because the hard evidence of a direct cause between Hepatitis C and tattoos has been elusive or hard to pin down. What they would need is to test people before they got a tattoo, and then again after, to finally determine if one caused the other. Because people are not routinely tested for Hepatitis until they are sick, or donating blood, we will continue to wonder. When a 30-year-old happily married man gets hepatitis and has never had a transfusion or any IV drugs, and has no other risk factors: It makes you wonder.

A University of Texas study found that 22% (1 in 5 people) of those studied with a tattoo also have Hepatitis C. Of the people without tattoos, only 3.5% (1 in 30) had Hepatitis C. That big difference is hard to figure out. The facts are important to know, even with the mystery behind them:

With Tattoo   ---   1 in 5 have Hepatitis C
Without Tattoo ---   1 in 30 have Hepatitis C

Heart Defects

There is also significant health risk if you have a heart defect from birth (congenital heart abnormality). A number of cardiologists were surveyed, and they recommend antibiotic use prior to and during a tattoo application. In addition, over three quarters of these child cardiologists recommend against tattoos altogether! If you have a congenital heart problem (or heart valve issues), you definitely need to consult your physician before getting a tattoo. Don't take a risk on the spur of the moment if you have such a condition. Plan ahead.

Malpractice Suits

The increase in tattoos has also caused an increase in law suits related to mishaps, bad outcomes, and unwanted infections. Tattoo parlors across the nation are seeing malpractice cases popping up from bad artistic outcomes to unwanted skin reactions to life threatening infections. Many of these cases, which are tried before sympathetic juries, are resulting in large cash judgments against the tattoo parlors.

Model Pamela Anderson reports getting Hepatitis C from sharing a needle while getting a tattoo with her then husband Tommy Lee. They have since broken up, and of course she now has two daily reminders to regret that relationship: a barbed wire tattoo and a deadly disease.

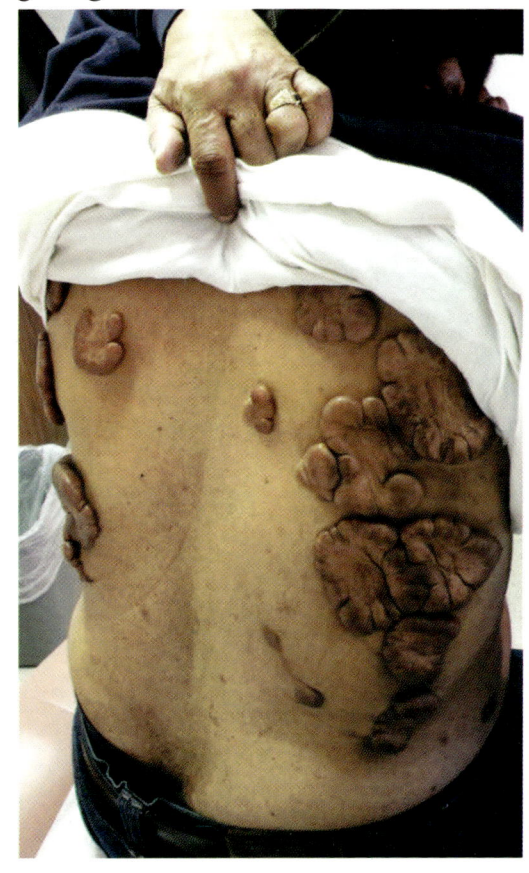

In an attempt to minimize the spread of these infections, the local health department inspects area tattoo parlors to ensure they have adequate protective measures, a clean environment, adequate sterilization techniques, new needles, clean procedures, and more. These inspections serve a vital purpose to help the tattoo parlors 'do the right thing'. Without someone keeping them honest, many more infections, due to cost cutting measures, would appear. The needles, the ink, the ink guns, alcohol, and time cleaning, all cost money and impact what a tattoo artist takes home at the end of the day. If you had one customer you're working on, and two waiting, wouldn't you move faster? And what would you compromise, the tattoo itself? or the clean up? We all know the final tattoo artistry is what brings future customers in, so that is a priority, but the clean-up may never be detected by the next unsuspecting customer.

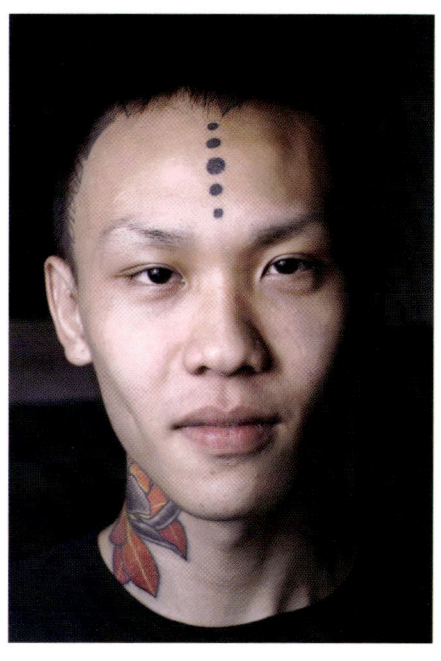

Obviously getting a tattoo in a run down, dark, dirty parlor is definitely a bad start to your tattoo experience.

The source of bacteria, or other infectious organisms, could begin with your skin. The skin naturally has hundreds of bacteria on a single spot at any given time. If the tattoo parlor is clean, and the needles are new, and the ink is sterile, you may still get an infection from bacteria inadequately cleaned from your own body. The outside of your skin, the epidermis, serves to protect the dermis, or layer below the epidermis. While the epidermis is very resistant to infection, the dermis is not. The introduction of just a few bacteria to the dermis can lead to an infection that could impact your life.

People considering tattoos should ensure that their tetanus and hepatitis B vaccines are up to date. At least if they are exposed, their vaccines can help protect them. There is currently no Hepatitis C vaccine. The real dilemma lies in individual reactions and experiences. Everyone's reaction to a tattoo differs. Just as spring allergies to pollen affect some people, and not others, your reaction to the needle process, ink, bacteria, healing, etc. can radically vary. There are a number of non-infectious skin reactions that differ from person to person.

Frankly, some people are good healers, and others get scars more easily. If you are the type to keep a scar (or the evidence of a scar) a very long time, the outcome of your tattoo will be

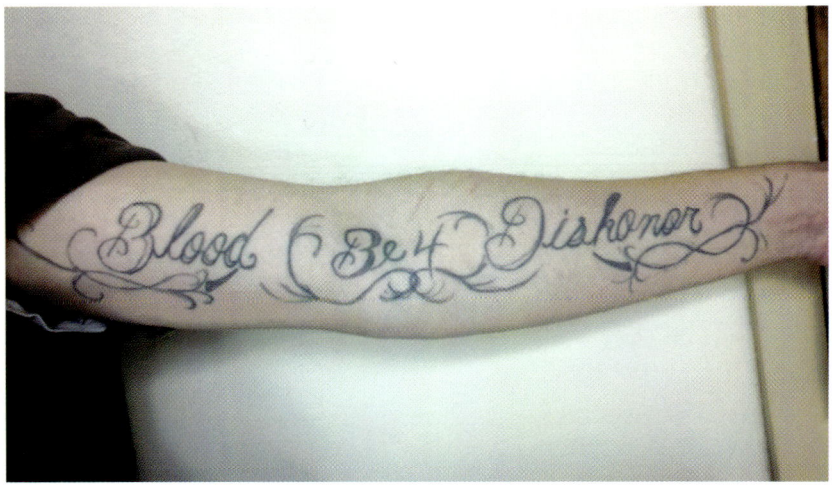

anybody's guess. Just read the fine print on the form in the tattoo parlor. . .they claim NO responsibility for bad outcomes. And by signing the form, you agree that you can't sue them for a bad outcome.

The worst outcomes include an antibiotic-

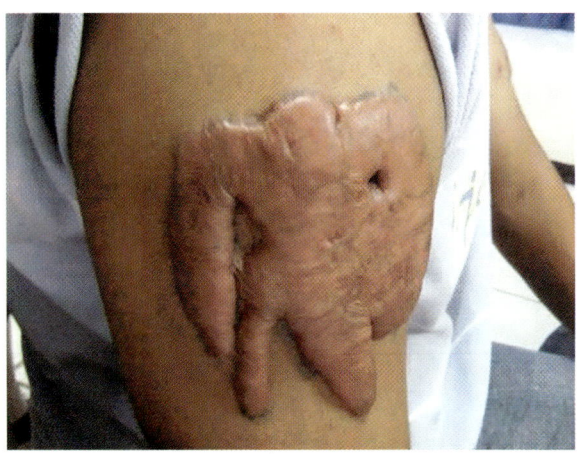

This keloid reaction is just one way the skin can react to injury.

resistant infection, or a keloid reaction. Everyone has heard of "flesh-eating bacteria" and if that gets into the dermis, the tattoo will heal in a disfiguring way. Others have a tendency to heal or scar in an abnormal way. This reaction is called keloid-ing, and the scar is called a keloid. Given the possibility of keloid-ing, everyone's first tattoo should be small and in a spot you can easily hide or cover for the rest of your life – just in case. Better safe than sorry.

So let's review: WHAT COULD GO WRONG?

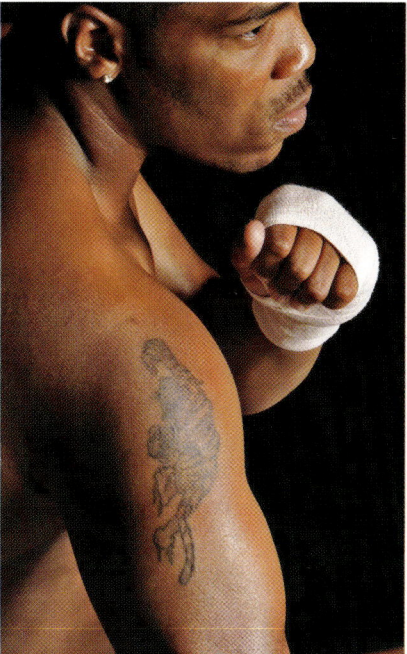

- Unclean tattoo area
- A bad tattoo artist
- Bad equipment/needles
- An unclean technique
- Heavy metal poisoning
- Keloid scarring
- Hepatitis B and C
- You can't donate blood for a year
- Tetanus
- Heart valve problems
- HIV/AIDS
- Staph infections
- Tattoo too big
- Can't join the military with an tattoo showing.
- Allergic reaction to certain inks
- You could be prevented from getting some x-rays

Question: What is that??
Answer: Bad Artist

- An outdated tattoo
- You might be viewed questionably by the college of choice
- You can't get the job you want
- You can't get a promotion
- It might be a stupid idea you regret because it was not thought through

Chapter 5: Your Future Career at Risk

Once in the work force, you will spend more time making money than any other endeavor, at least 8 hours a day, plus the commute! Your ability to get, and then keep, a job will rest on a number of factors. Among them are:

- ***Are you a good worker?***
- ***Are you reliable?***
- ***Will you show up on time?***
- ***Do you represent the company well?***

"Representing the company" includes wearing clean neat clothes and a reasonable hairstyle, but it also means what, if any, tattoos you have, where they are, and what does this body art suggests about the worker.

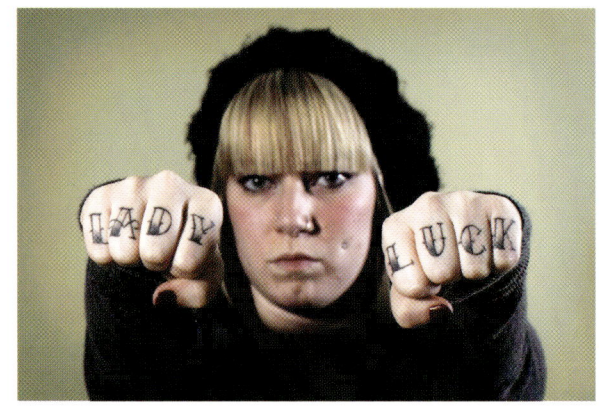

One waiter in a restaurant, because of his past boxing interest as a youth, tattooed L-E-T-H-A-L on the knuckles of his right hand and W-E-A-P-O-N on the left (and no, he didn't have six fingers on each hand!). When he was shaking his boss's hand at the interview, the boss delayed hiring him until he could confirm that he wasn't a felon. As he handed food to diners, they might think the food was poisoned, so he had created a method of holding his hands so they could not easily read them. Essentially, what he did to get attention as a teen boxer haunted him daily, it greatly affected his ability to earn money. When he finally met his future wife, she thought for months that he might beat her, too.

A nurse at a hospital tells how as a late teen she was in love with Steve, her first boyfriend. Her love was so deep and loyal that she had his name tattooed on her neck so her commitment could be seen by all who met her. Steve left, as almost all first boyfriends do, because she was too "crazy for him." She is still left to explain, 10 years later, why she did such a thing as get a tattoo showing undying love for someone who, when all is said and done, did not feel the same way about her. In the meantime, she is in a turtleneck sweater from September to April and a fashionable scarf during the summer. What seemed like a passionate act of love and commitment is now just a daily reminder of a stupid mistake. In this complicated world, preconception or pre-judgment is very common. Don't put yourself at a disadvantage by putting a tattoo in a overly obvious location like the hands, lower arms, neck and of course, the face. People may make the wrong snap judgment about you.

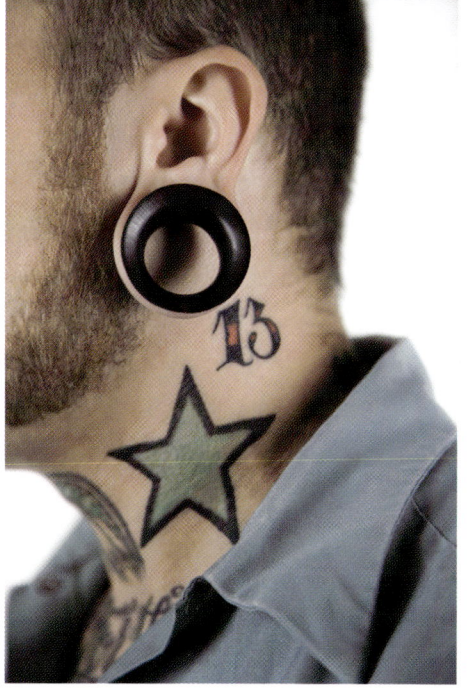

For whatever reason, desperate people have begun tattooing their face with an array of graffiti, profanity, or curse words. They wrongfully believe this act of expression will be overlooked when times get hard, and they need to get a job that pays more than minimum wage. This is a foolish risk. The latest craze is to tattoo famous rappers' signs on the face. This is the most stupid, irresponsible fad ever envisioned. It can't last, but unfortunately, the tattoo will.

> *A young man applied for a lucrative job in sales. It involved taking an employment exam and required many interviews. After he did extremely well on the exam and impressed the last interviewer, his future boss proceeded to offer him the job! As they extended hands for a congratulatory handshake, the boss noticed a tattoo on the back of his hand, and ended the interview with "I'm sorry."*

The story above may be unfair and discriminatory, but it is also a fact of life. A completely competent person can lose a job opportunity simply because of something as trivial as a tattoo or body piercing. The military (Army, Navy, etc.) <u>will not</u> allow you to apply with an "obvious" tattoo (neck, face, hands, etc.).

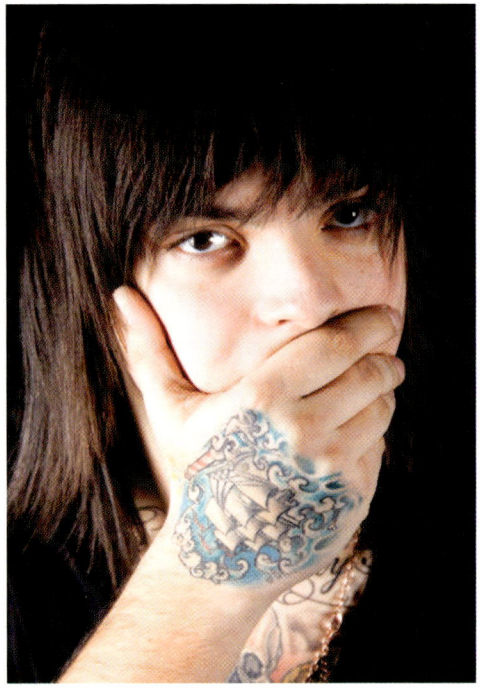

Just because everyone you know has a tattoo or piercing doesn't mean it is accepted everywhere. When going to an interview for a job that involves dealing with the public, ALWAYS conceal any body art.

So to be fair, unless your plan is to be a tattoo artist, or a rock band member, or a motorcycle repair shop owner, or something along those lines, keep your body art easily concealed, at least through the interview process, and probably indefinitely into the future.

You probably should NOT have a visible tattoo if you want to be:

- President, Governor, Senator, or other politician
- A social worker, or other job working with the public
- A physician or a nurse in a leadership position
- A receptionist, secretary, or clerk
- A salesperson
- A military soldier, officer or operative.
- A model or beauty queen
- A lead actress or actor
- A minister or priest
- A judge, counselor, or arbitrator
- A TV announcer, moderator, or host
- Promoted to a position of leadership in a company

You probably can have a visible tattoo if you want to be:

- A cosmetologist
- A barber or stylist
- An artist , painter, or sculptor
- An appliance repair person
- A mechanic
- An exotic dancer
- A musician
- An actor or actress playing villains
- A rapper, band musician, or travel band support (stage hand lighting, etc.)
- A professional athlete not planning to work on TV or in business after your career
- A radio announcer or DJ

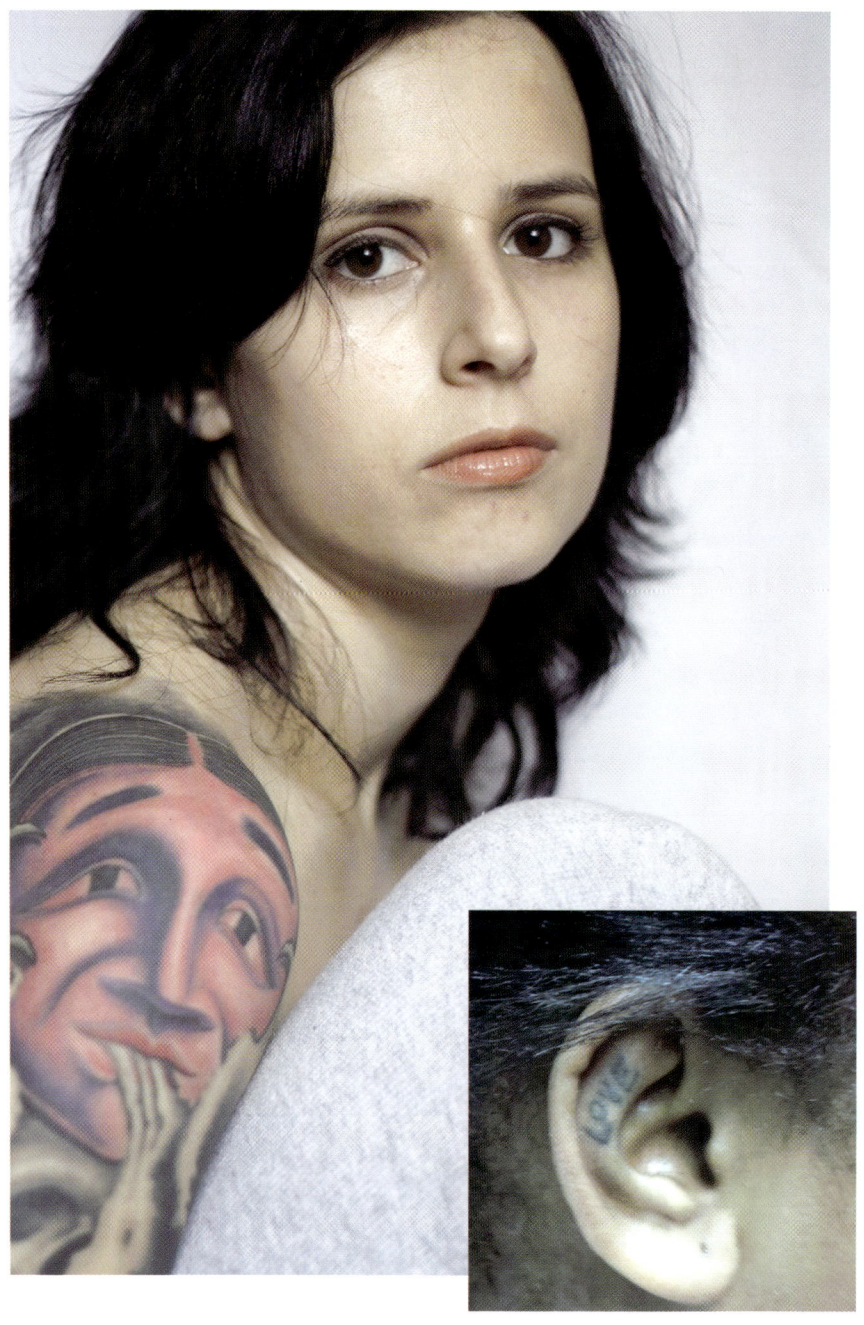

Chapter 6: "But all of my friends have one!"

"If all of your friends jumped off a bridge, would you do that too?" As crazy as that question is, the answer for many teenagers might be: "Yes, I would jump off a bridge if all of my friends did." Come on, now. The pressure to be accepted in today's society is enormous, but use some common sense.. Hair styles, clothing styles, and social habits are frequently pushed upon the impressionable. Not following a fad, like tattoos, will take a great strength of character.

Peer pressure is the unspoken influence to conform. Much of what our society appreciates is the result of peer pressure and conformity.

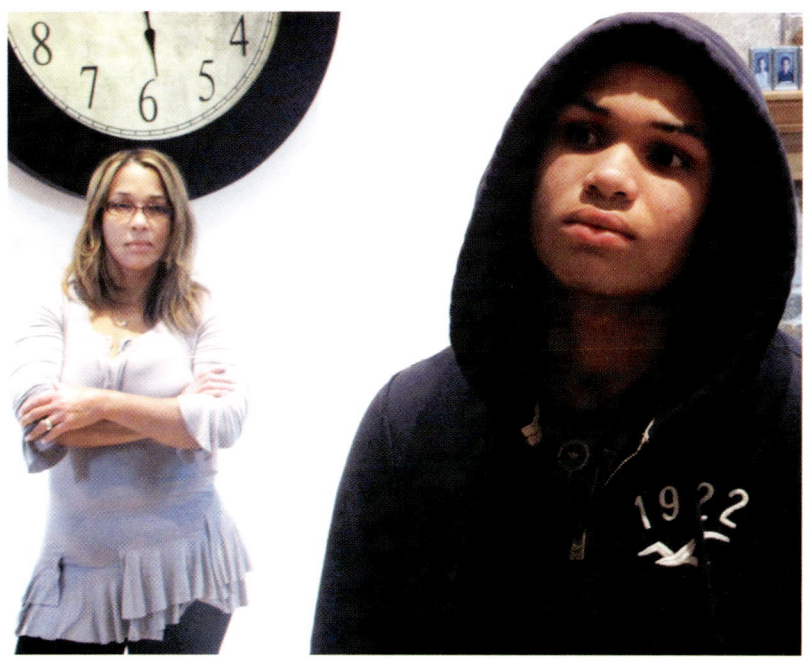

Imagine if you are on a flat country road. You can see for miles in every direction and no one, no other car, no police, nothing is around. You come to a stop sign where one road crosses another. The vast majority of Americans will stop (or at least slow down significantly) as they cross that intersection. That is done because of peer pressure, training, and habit.

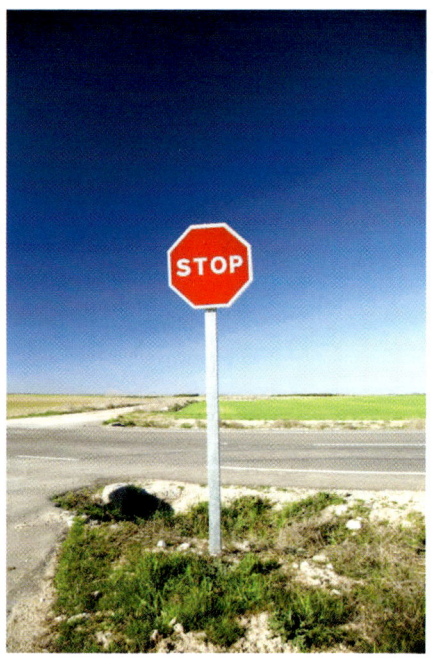

Doing what your friends are doing . . .

- ✓ **like wearing similar hair styles**
- ✓ **listening to the same music**
- ✓ **buying the most popular shoes**
- ✓ **joining a gang, fraternity, or sorority**
- ✓ **having multiple children out of marriage**

are all the result of peer pressure.

None of these actions come innately: They have to be learned from the larger body of society. What we accept as a civilization is also dictated by peer pressure. Today, mainstream "easy listening" music consists of Michael Jackson, Earth, Wind and Fire, and the Beatles. Their music is heard in department stores, hospital waiting rooms, and elevators across the country. Thirty years ago, this was fringe music absolutely NOT accepted in the those locations; instead Perry Como and Frank Sinatra were the standards. Because of societal acceptance, comfort, and peer pressure, what is accepted has changed significantly.

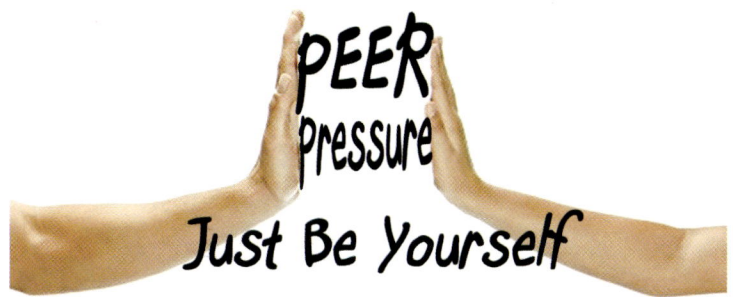

The logical next question is . . . in twenty years will tattoos be a universally accepted form of personal expression? The answer is a definite "maybe." But what will more likely be accepted will be self expression through creativity, not a trendy Gucci Mane ice cream cone, or a Sponge-Bob cartoon; no one will know what either is by then.

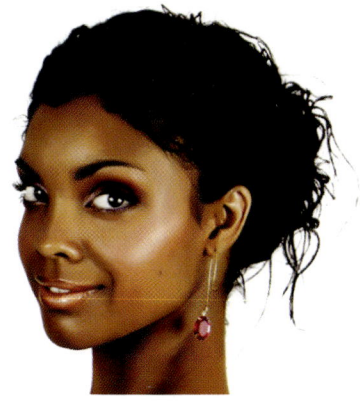

The perfect example of a universally accepted body art is a woman's pierced ear. Four out of 5 women have their ear lobes pierced, and this practice is completely accepted by nearly everyone. In fact, if a woman doesn't wear earrings at a formal event or an interview, that could be seen as unusual. This accepted practice hasn't always been in vogue. Years ago aristocratic woman "of class" never wore earrings. Only sailors, pirates, and gypsies were seen with ear piercings or earrings. With the passing of time, more women were getting ear jewelry to the extent that "everyone" was doing it. In fact, most women get their ears pierced as very young girls, or even as babies.

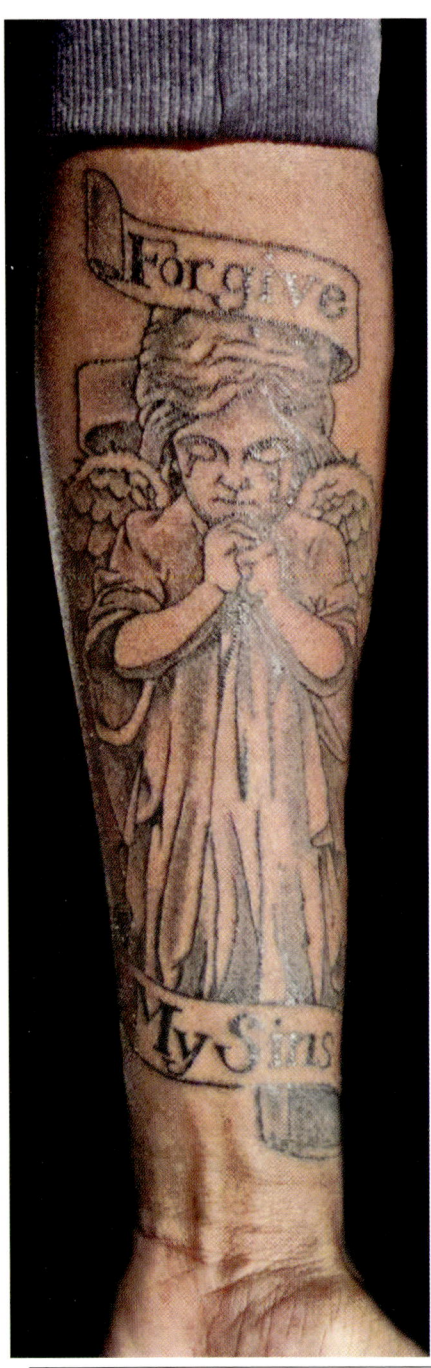

So almost "all your friends" have a tattoo, and you want one too? Ask yourself why? Do you want one for your own benefit, or do you want one to show to others? If you had one and didn't show it, or admit to it, would that bother you? That's how you tell peer pressure from personal desire. And these are important things to think about.

If you want a nice car to pick up women, or impress your friends, that's peer pressure. If you get a nice car and only admire it while driving on an empty road by yourself, that's desire. If you want a tattoo for your own enjoyment, it really doesn't need to be in an obvious location, and therefore limit your career options dramatically. If your tattoo is really for other people's enjoyment, shock, or benefit, you need to closely examine the motivation, your self-esteem, and the long term value of that endeavor. Think about how you really want to be viewed by others.

The moral of this discussion is that peer pressure is not necessarily bad, or dysfunctional: It is merely a fact of life. Knowing what drives you to do the things you do is part of maturity. Making a decision about your life and body that is permanent **requires** some inward thought and reflection. As Shakespeare said "to thine own self be true" or recognize what motivates you, and occasionally "take the road less traveled," as poet Robert Frost put it, that unique decision might make "all the difference."

Where to put your tattoo?

If this book doesn't convince you not to get a tattoo -- and you are already positive that you want a permanent reminder of your first love, or first born, or first loss -- then the second most important decision is the location of your tattoo. There are multiple locations on the body that are popular: the top of the arm, the small of the back, the buttock, an ankle, and so on. How people decide is an issue of personal preference. Usually, the more dramatic (first love, first death, etc.), the more prominent the location chosen. A boyfriend who dies in the Army or in a motor vehicle accident may get a neck tattoo in his tragic honor. A simple tattoo fad adoption move may just warrant Mickey Mouse on the back of a shoulder, or a ornamental design on the small of the back.

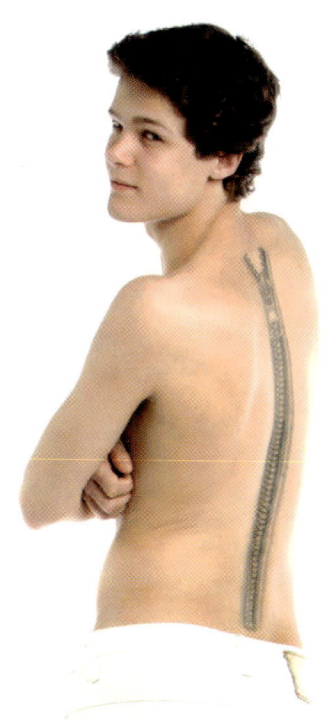

Men tend to choose the macho slave designs (the barbed wire around the upper arm) or the devil's favorite, the skull and crossbones on the forearm. When you are single, these can be a sign of great manhood or machismo. Once married with children, however, the symbols become a sign of "what once was."

If you have a cross on your chest, you'll see it, your close family and friends will see it, but co-workers, employees, and the public almost never will. There will be no impact to your career choices and no pre-judgment by the public. A tattoo on your forearm will be seen sooner or later at work, and things may change. . .Most importantly, though, your feelings about your tattoo may change with the passing of time.

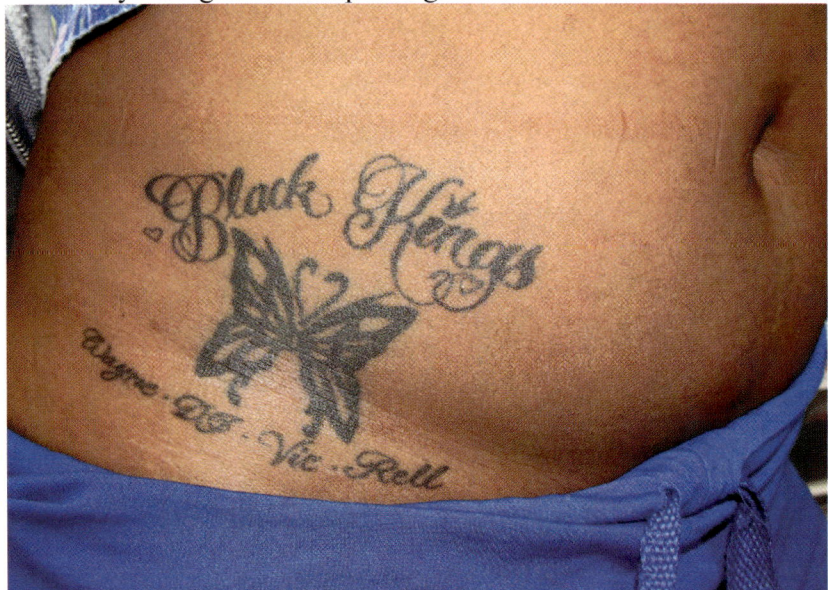

The moral here is to choose an easily concealed spot. Why? Because you WILL have to explain your decision to get the tattoo, and you will only have to explain the concealed ones to the few people who ultimately see them. Tattoos on your neck, calves, forearms, wrists, and ankles will have to be explained to future employers, future spouses, and future children. While these might serve as conversation-starters, the novelty will fade and the conversation will be as unenviable as telling the story of how you lost an eye (which usually begins with. . ."I hope you didn't notice.")

On the positive side, a tattoo could easily be placed on the upper thigh or buttock, and be only seen in bathing suits and daisy dukes. Getting a tattoo in these seldom-seen places is akin to having a scar there. No worrying about who sees it. . .and if someone does sees it: Who cares?`

The main motivation to get a tattoo, other than most of your friends already have one, is to personalize yourself, but do it in a personal way, use an easily concealed location.

A loss in your life

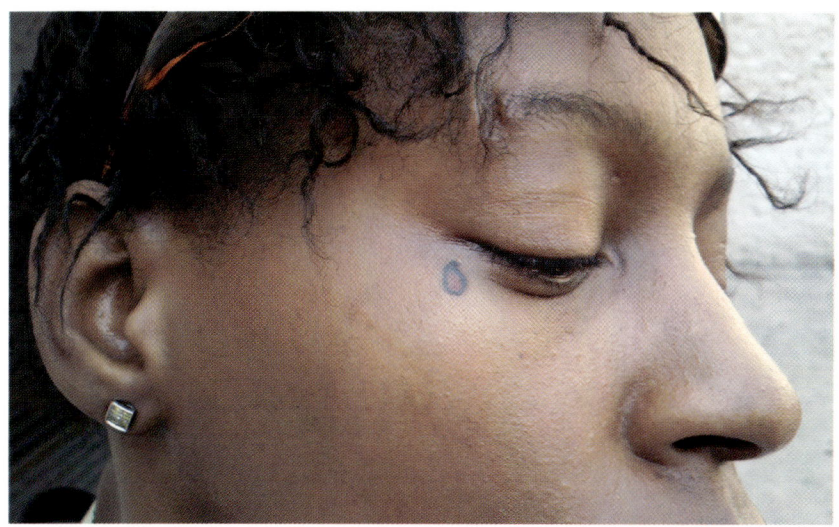

> *"My mother died, and I wanted to show the world my grief in a big and permanent way, so I got tear drops tattooed on my face below my eyes."* *As I got older and saw all of my friends' parents die, and how they handled the situation with grace and dignity, I felt stupid showing my tears and fragility to others."*

What this individual also doesn't know is that each teardrop tattooed on the face is a popular gang sign of the number of people they killed. Imagine the misunderstandings that could arise from this innocent gesture of love.

We will all lose loved ones, and although the loss is deep and scarring, there is no need to further scar the situation with a memorial tattoo. Death is a part of life, and you can and will remember your loved ones without the extra reminder.

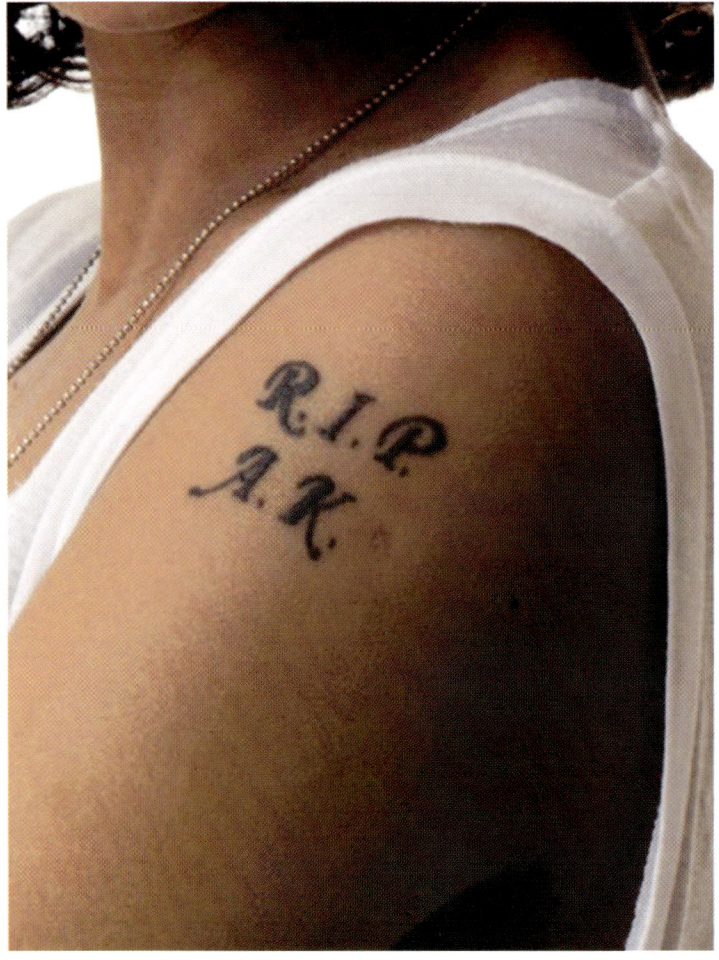

Chapter 7: "Permanent," but Changing. . .

So the tattoo is permanent right? That means I have to look at it the rest of my life. . .right? Right. But here's the part I've left out until now: Tattoos change over time. They fade, sag, and run like the design on old wall paper. You read that right: fading, sagging, running. Have you ever seen a paint color or

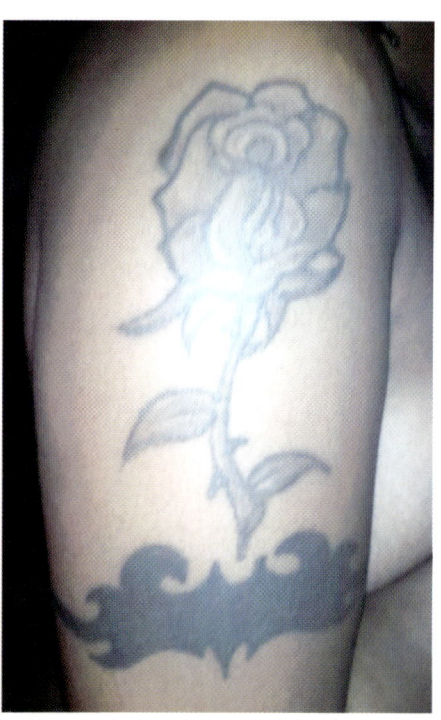

The RED has left this tattoo, it now just grey.

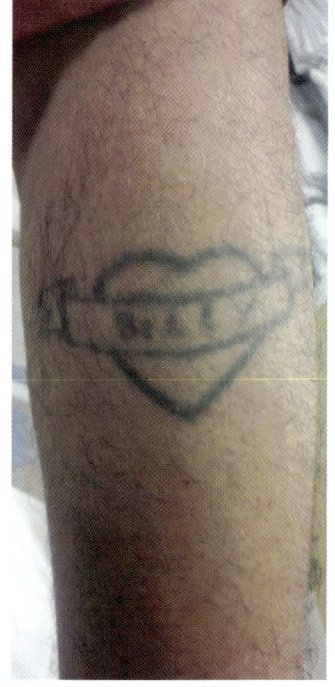

wall paper with a horrible color or design? Well, it wasn't like that when it was new. At first, it was vibrant, crisp, defined, and interesting. Frequently after 10 years or so, it has lost its vivid colors to faded shades, its crisp definition yields to a hazy design many hesitate to define or figure out. Don't be taken by surprise. That may happen to your tattoo.

Tattoos stretch, sag, and distort, depending on where they are located on the body. A stomach tattoo may start as a sexy emblem and morph over time to a huge eyesore. Tattoos that have been exposed to the sun also have a large amount of color distortion 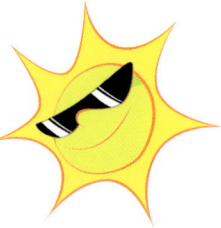 over time. If the tattoo is placed in an area with increased 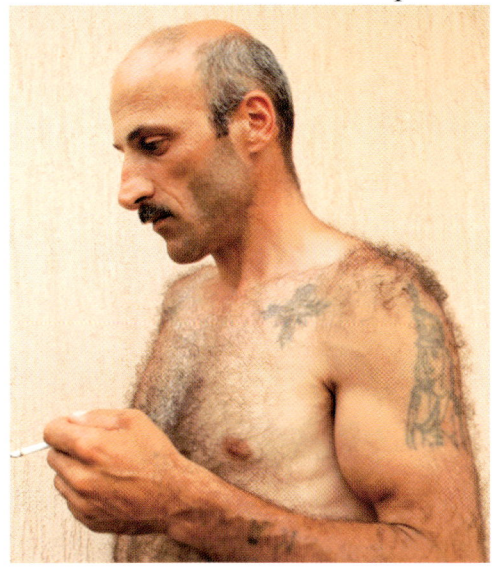 weight loss, the tattoo will distort and wrinkle and the image will definitely change. People cannot predict how their own shape may change. A simple nine-month pregnancy can drastically and permanently change a tattoo for the worse. While the design in the small of your back may be sexy on a bikini-clad 22 year old, it looks dated on a 50 year old, and even ridiculous on a 70 year old. Have you ever seen an older person with long eye lashes, and gobs of makeup, and thought "oh my word, what was she thinking?" The answer is she was, and is, thinking the same things she was months and years ago.

Almost all people with tattoos report a significant change in the tattoo from when it was new. For whatever reason, some tattoos fade faster in some people and less so in others. The colors can also look as if they're running, blurring, or smudging. Actually the cells in your body are trying to take the pigment away, and are ultimately unsuccessful. This can occur with any tattoo, but seems to happen more in the face and neck with cosmetic tattoos (permanent eyeliner, eyebrows applications, etc.).

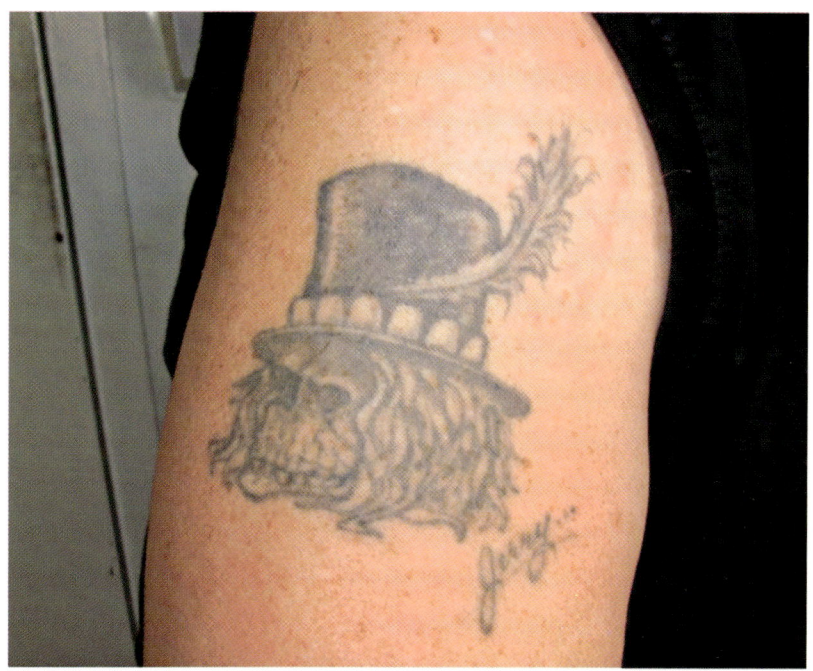

Note how much this tattoo has faded after 10 years.

There are also certain colors that give more trouble with fading than others. Generally the colors red, orange, yellow, and bright purple will fade over time, while the blue and black tattoo will hold somewhat better. The main cause of fading tattoos is sun exposure, more specifically, ultraviolet light. Bright vibrant colors in a tattoo may fade as fast as just one week with sun exposure, so

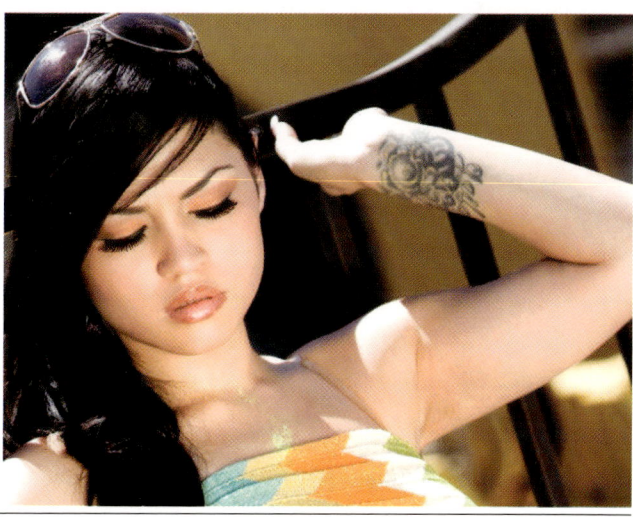

choosing a covered/hidden location will help maintain the beauty if you want a bold color.

Choosing a first design with colors in mind (avoiding colors that fade, or picking a location that is not sun exposed), and keeping the size small so that you can see what your skin does in response to a tattoo is the <u>smartest</u> and <u>safest</u> approach.

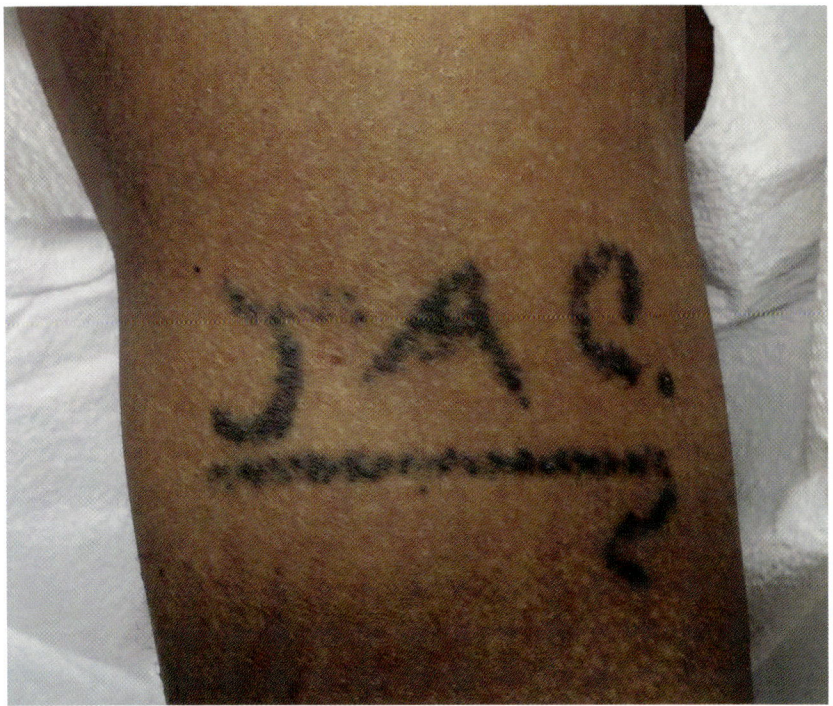

This 'home-made' tattoo was done with
a straight pen and ink. One stick at a time.

Chapter 8: Do *NOT* Get These Tattoos

When considering body art, it is best to take advice from people with experience. In other words, listen to people who already have tattoos and piercing, and listen to their advice. By and large the people who end up happy with their tattoos are the ones who use creativity. They usually design the art and then describe the final effect they are looking for to the artist. Looking through a book for tattoo ideas is a bad start. Think about your personality, thoughts, and aspirations and imagine how body art will improve on them. It is a fact that body art is not for everyone. Have you ever noticed a tattoo that seemed perfectly suited for the wearer? On the other hand, how many times have you seen a tattoo that just looked stupid, or a man or woman who impacted their overall looks negatively by a poorly thought-out tattoo?

How often do you see a tattoo on regular people (excluding the internet and TV) that really adds to their beauty? I am guessing your answer. . . "not that often." The reason is that those people that put thought into their tattoo and how it will mesh with their body type and style are far more successful with the final product. Not all clothes complement all wearers. A single dress can look great on one wearer and horrible on another. This is why we "try on" suits and shirts because although we have chosen the correct size, the "fit" may not be appropriate.

What goes along with the theme of having body art "complement" the wearer is throwing out entire categories of tattoos for most people. The basic theme is to make your tattoo as unique as the body it is going on. Avoid the tattoo that looks cool on someone else. Instead, be creative and personalize the tattoo to your interests, ambitions, and beliefs. Remember whatever future profession you want should impact your decision. If you intend to be a model, actor, or celebrity, tattoos are definitely out! If you want to be in the military, FBI, CIA, or CSI (despite what you see on TV), tattoos are out! So don't kill your dreams before you even got started on a path to success.

ANY TATTOO ON YOUR FACE OR NECK

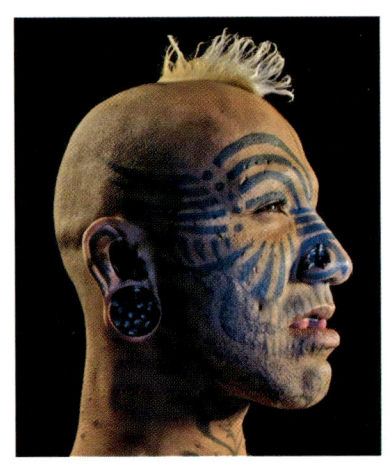

Unless it is for medical reasons, a tattoo on your face or neck is a bad idea . . .period.

YOUR GIRLFRIEND OR BOYFRIEND'S NAME

In the heat of true love, most people search for a meaningful way to express their deep-seated feelings for another. Saying "I love you" seems to fall short. Sailors and soldiers have consistently chosen MOM as a safe tattoo selection while away at sea or war, but even

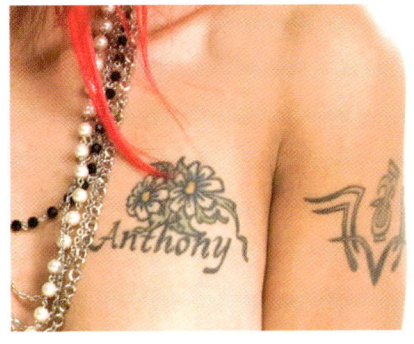

they rarely tattooed a love interests name on their arm. While your "endless love" may endure (despite statistics that show it won't), it is always a bad idea to tattoo a mate's name on your body. Setting aside the fact that the relationship might end, and you will be left explaining the persistent tattoo to others (and quietly to yourself), the so-called act of love actually has a paradoxical effect on the relationship. In some cases, the tattoo is seen as a manipulation. The thoughts that "I am owned by you" or "you own me, and no one else" can instill a sense of smothering or binding to a relationship that frequently hasn't been *mutually* agreed upon. It would be smarter to affirm your love of "LOVE" or "Commitment" in the form of a small easily hidden tattoo.

A CHINESE SYMBOL

The reason for not getting the Chinese symbols falls in the "avoid a fad" category. Certainly, if you speak Chinese, are of Chinese heritage, or love martial arts, then you can still use this overused theme, but if you (or others) have to do research to determine the meaning, it's a bad idea. Besides, you might accidentally put something "stupid" in Chinese on your body.

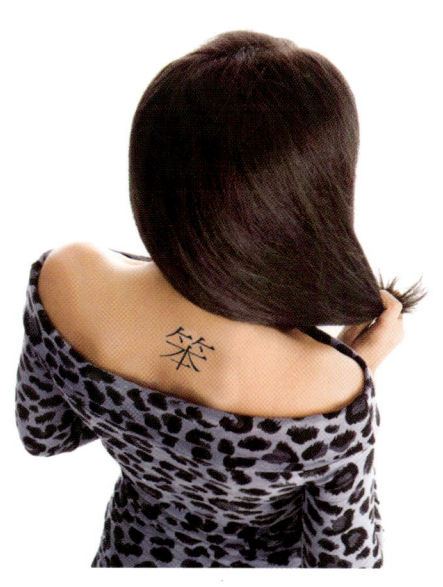

BARBED WIRE

Wow, that's really tough! If you really want to impress

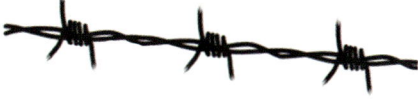

someone, wrap a real barbed wire around your arm. The first guys to do it were cool and creative. Now it's just unimaginative and repetitive.

A CARTOON FIGURE

While SpongeBob is funny, and I doubt he will be going away any time soon, it also is too trendy and fleeting for your body.

Design your own cartoon personalized to you. Imagine if you designed a cartoon for yourself, had it tattooed on your arm, and then the guy down the street put your tattoo on his arm, too. Create your own stuff.

A POP-CULTURE REFERENCE

That would be something that is hot now and gone in five years, like the peace sign, or "Yes we can." Please be a little more creative with your permanent art. Don't use pop culture references. Otherwise, you will quickly look behind the times.

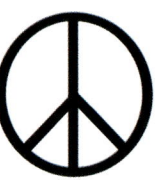

A FACE

Your body should have only one face. . . yours. More than one face on a body is "just creepy." If the person is still alive, they will change. What if you had Michael Jackson at age 15 tattooed (and many did), and then Michael at 45 showed up. . .two totally different pictures. What if you were an avid Buffalo Bills fan and had OJ Simpson (an incredible running back in the 1970's) tattooed on your arm. Twenty years later you now have a generally hated convict prominently displayed on your arm.

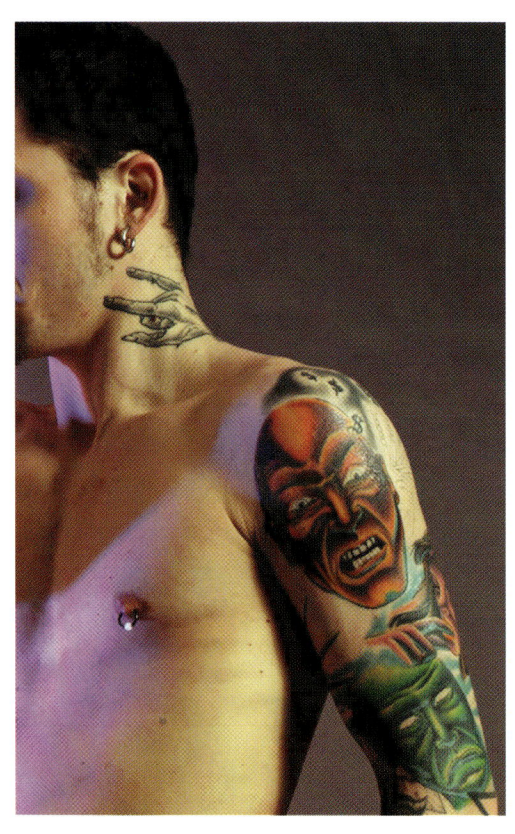

A SUPER HERO EMBLEM

Avoid this unless you are the actual super hero. It's okay for Clark Kent, although the tattooist would have trouble penetrating that steel, but the design is too short-sighted for earthlings.

Again, the reason these DON'Ts get their own chapter is because these are the impulsive tattoos that people refuse to put thought into before they get them. It's easy to copy someone else (who actually may have put thought into it), but the true purpose of successful tattoos is to have something complementary to your body, your spirit, and your mind. You can't do what other people do, and have it work.

An extremely sexy tattoo in the small of a woman's back may work for her, but look bad on you because:

1.) your back's anatomy is not suitable for a tattoo;
2.) your skin tone doesn't match the ink colors chosen;
3.) the design doesn't suit your personality or beliefs;
4.) the tattoo artist isn't as good, or not having as good a day;
5.) your system rejects and blurs/fades the design.

The worse decision you can make is to pick a tattoo based on how good it looks on another person. Spend the appropriate amount of time selecting the tattoo just right for you, or wait a little. . .and not get one at all.

Chapter 9: Tattoo removal

From a medical standpoint, tattoos are, and should be, considered permanent. The ink is put in a place that does not renew and 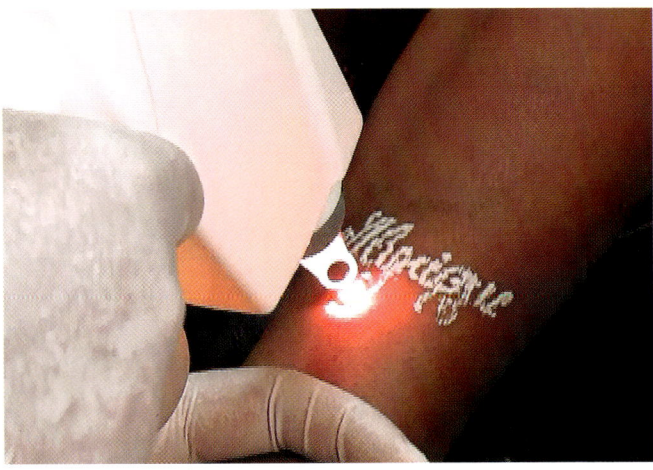 therefore will remain for the rest of your life. With all the "mistakes" related to tattoos (bad artist, bad design, wrong color, wrong size, wrong name, wrong place, and so on) there has developed a new multimillion dollar industry called ***tattoo removal.***

The people who show up for tattoo removal vary from men to women (although most are women) and young to old (most are younger). They all have a common set of characteristics:

1. They desperately want their tattoo removed (and without a scar);

2. They have the money to pay for the removal;

3. They clearly believe the pain of removal is less than the pain of having to look at the tattoo the rest of their life.

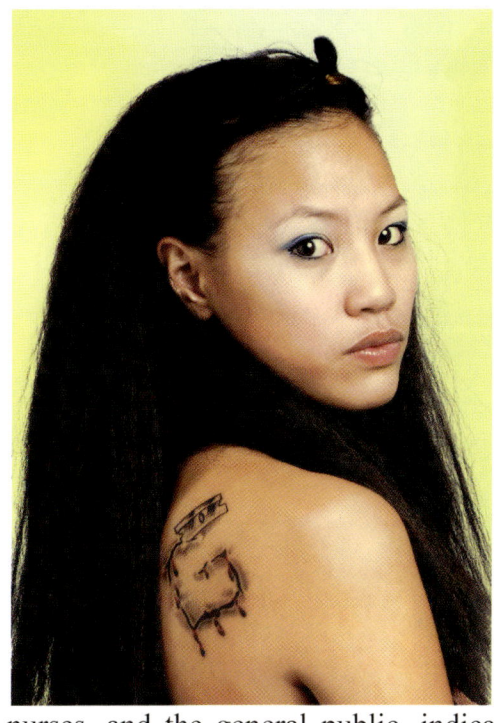

A study looked at the actual reasons people gave for finally coming to the clinic and scheduling laser tattoo removal. While women tended to be more deliberate and thoughtful before getting a tattoo, that is, they did more research and were generally more sure about the decision; some found over time that they "experience some negative, stereotypic responses to the tattoos from their fathers, physicians, registered nurses, and the general public, indicating possession risk" they hadn't considered (nor could they have) in advance. In short, they didn't expect the reaction they got, nor did they expect their own reaction to the unexpected reaction, so they decided to remove the tattoo. These more educated, career-minded women simply could not afford to be pre-judged as impulsive and whimsical in a competitive business environment that values level-headed decisiveness.

High Expectations can lead to Great Disappointment

This study also found that people's expectations of the final outcome of tattoo removal were unusually high. Many thought the tattoo could be removed completely without any evidence of its prior existence. This is generally NOT the case. There is "usually" some degree of scarring after tattoo removal that an observant person can detect. The success of tattoo removal hinges on a number of factors, many of which are completely out of your control, but there are some guidelines.

All agree that the success of tattoo removal varies with:
- the size of the tattoo (smaller is easier)
- the skin tone (lighter skin is better)
- the age of the tattoo (newer tattoos are easier to remove)
- the age and healing ability of the individual (younger is better)
- professionally done versus homemade (non-professional tattoos are easier to remove)
- the colors in the tattoo (more vivid colors are tougher to remove)
- the laser used.

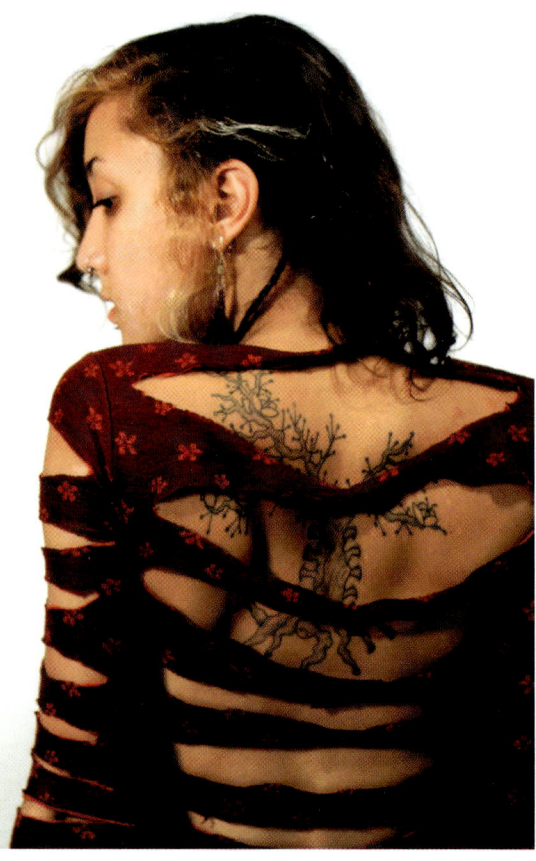

The vast majority of the people in this study (75%) had gotten the tattoo (they now want removed) during their adolescence (age 12 to 19). Also of note, a majority (42%) were happy with the tattoo result at first, while 27% were initially unhappy. The remaining 31% that aren't sure how they felt at first, are sure now: They want the tattoo removed.

When people are specifically asked why they want their tattoo removed, fatigue is the answer. They are tired of hiding it. Most have developed a wide variety of methods to mask the tattoo, and will use clothing, make-up, Band-Aids, and jewelry. And despite their best efforts, the tattoo is still detected (and judged) more frequently than they would like. While these same individuals will strongly deny that they were ordered, or made to, remove the tattoo, they obviously felt a pressure, or compulsion to do it. Tattoo removal is not an impulse move. It takes four to eight (or more) sessions separated by weeks and months of healing and wound care. While the tattoo can be placed in an evening, its removal is a much more arduous and time-consuming task, and one that takes ongoing

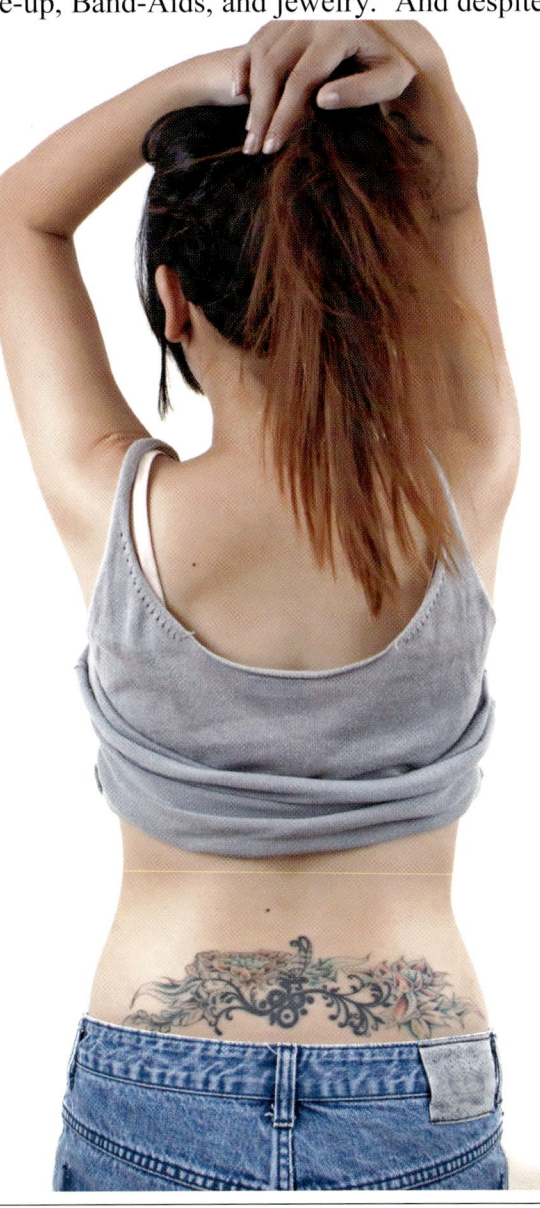

conviction and resolve.

When psychologists analyze the motivations for tattoo removal, the main drive is a "distancing from the past." Many of those who want it removed experienced very strong emotions 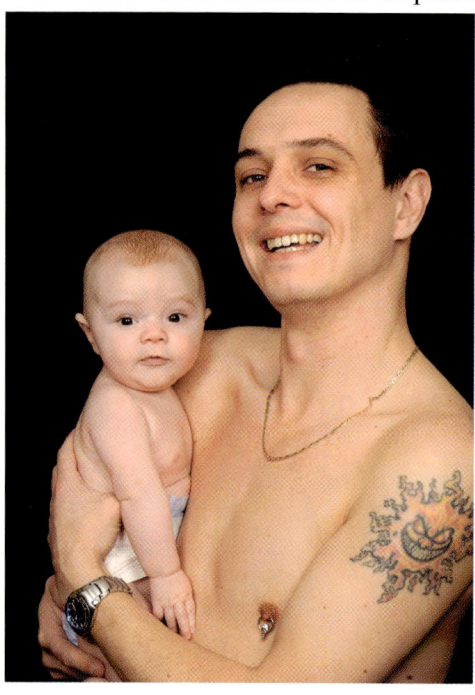 when obtaining the tattoo: love, grief, rebellion, isolation, anger, and so on. Over time, the tattoo is a daily visual reminder of that time, that person, and those intense feelings. Eventually, the person wants to distance himself or herself from that era and those feelings, and the only way is by removing the tattoo.

Others get a different perspective on life when they bring a child into the world. Parents of any age are more thoughtful about the consequences of decisions they make ... including body art. They are conscious of the example they set, and ultimately how they are viewed by their growing children. Essentially the rebellion of youth is replaced by a need to be viewed in a responsible manner. A radical tattoo or piercing is much less important.

It would be interesting to see if the people who don't go for tattoo removal are the opposite. Did they NOT get their tattoo in association with strong feelings? Do they NOT try to hide their tattoos? Do they truly NOT care what other people think? Or is it simply that they don't have the money or commitment to tolerate the removal process?

Researchers have also found that when career-minded people think long and hard about getting a tattoo, and comparison shop as it relates to design, tattoo artist, and tattoo shop, they tend to be happier with their tattoo, spend less time covering it up, and are less likely to have it removed later. Adolescents' getting a tattoo without careful consideration of its impact on their lives is by far the most common regret surfacing in tattoo removal clinics across the country. Education is the answer.

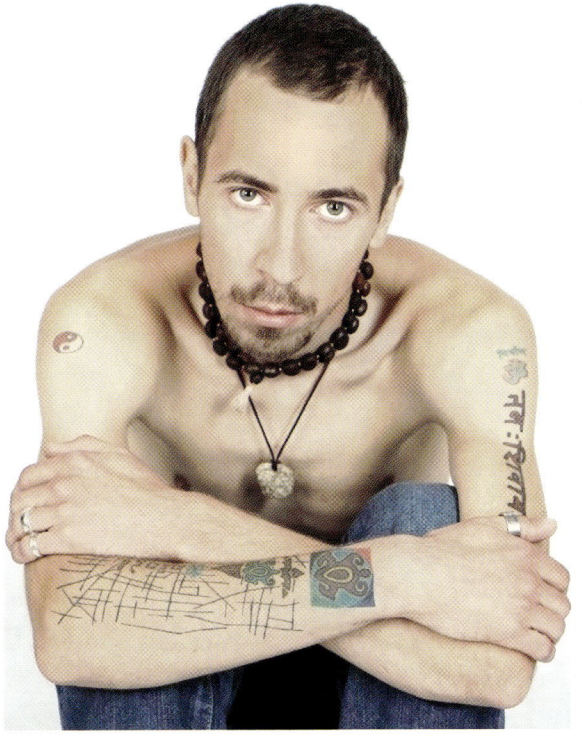

Beyond these major psychological motivations, laser removal clinics also see a trend in what specifically their patrons wanted removed. Area researchers surveyed laser removal specialists, tallied their clients' characteristics, and published these results. Note that these tattoo removal winners also closely coincide with the earlier Tattoo DON'Ts in this book.

1. **Lower Back Tattoos**: AKA "tramp stamp." It's cute on a thin 22 year old, but after age 30, a large number of women find they really don't want it anymore.

2. **Comic Book Superheroes:** Like the tramp stamp, guys in their twenties tend to still idolize heroes, but when they enter their 30's and beyond, these hero emblems begin to make the men look retarded.

3. **Barbed Wire**: It seems women as they get older go to more formal functions socially and with their business. The barbed wire on their arm kills the gown effect.

4. **Chinese Symbols**: The stereotypical "I want to be original" tattoo, has become commonplace. People are either having the symbol incorporated into a new tattoo, or removing it altogether. Do you really know what your symbol actually means?

5. **Names:** Don't do it. Don't do it! This expression of love is sure to kill the relationship.

This list assumes the art, technique, and outcome were all acceptable. They just got tired of the style (or the statement). A host of inferior tattoos find their way to the tattoo removal clinic as well, and they tend to go much sooner when it is easier to remove.

Tattoo Removal Options

There are a number of accepted tattoo removal processes. In all cases, the tattoo removal process is painful, scarring, and requires multiple treatments.
- ✓ Laser Removal (burn it off)
- ✓ Chemical (burn it off)
  - ○ Trichloroacetic Acid
- ✓ Abrasion (sand it off)
- ✓ Excision (cut it out)
- ✓ Variot Tattoo Removal (tattoo it off with chemicals)
- ✓ Bleaching/Fading Creams (many can cause cancer)

People have even had their tattoos *cut out*, rather than bear a daily reminder of a childish mistake. Laser therapy has progressed, but the process still involves repeated burns to the skin, healing , and then repeated burns. Big tattoos take longer to remove, and lighter skin works much better than darker skin.

Other ways to remove tattoos include chemical burns (as opposed to laser burns), and literally sanding or scrapping off the tattoo.

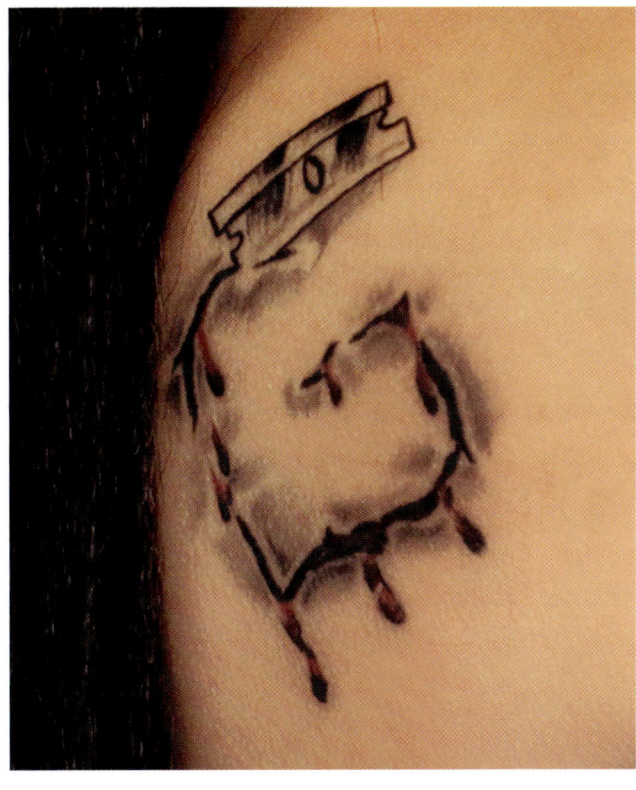

The tattoo removal process has to disrupt the dermis in order for the body to remove the dye. When a more dramatic wound than a tattoo occurs, the body can gradually clear out all debris (and ink) and heal. The important issue here is: How well do you heal? Some people heal scars completely with no residual skin changes, others heal and leave evidence of the trauma (a scar). If you are a "good healer" tattoo removal by laser or chemical burn may be a good option. If you heal and leave keloid scars, and obvious burn marks, it may be a better option to keep the tattoo. The tattoo removal people CANNOT guarantee the outcome regardless of what they say. Read the patient/client authorization sheet they ask you to sign before the procedure. It will specify what they are promising. What a person says can be misremembered, but what you sign is defensible in court. READ the contract and consider what it says (and doesn't say) before you go for a procedure. By fully understanding the tattoo removal process, the healing time, the number of visits, the "usual outcome," and other options, your expectations will be more realistic, and your outcome much more acceptable.

For whatever reason, professional tattoos are harder to remove than homemade/amateur/house party tattoos. Maybe they are not as deep or consistent, but the simple fact that whatever mode of removal you use, a professionally done tattoo will go away more slowly. This does NOT mean you should go amateur when getting a tattoo; it's just a fact of the industry. If you made a horrible tattoo party mistake, you may be blessed with a better outcome if you have it removed.

Laser Removal

By far the most popular, and most say the best, form of tattoo removal is laser removal. A simple review of the Internet will reveal a massive number of places offering the treatment. The choices are so plentiful, it is hard to narrow down the options. Your best choice is to find a physician who sub-specializes in laser removal, or to choose an organization that does laser removal all day. Try to avoid the places with lasers that do hair removal and tummy 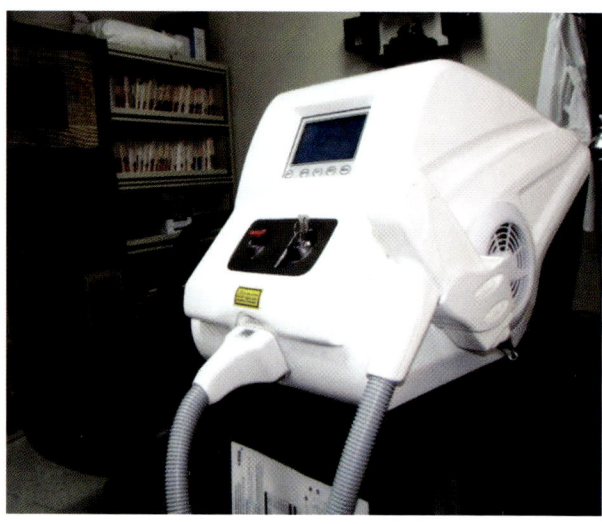 tucks, and Botox, and on and on. The company you want needs good experience with tattoo removal (and maybe one other thing). Ask to review "before and after" photos of their previous work.

Ask about the laser. There are a number of lasers with a different element base (Argon vs. Carbon-based), varying frequencies, different responses to tattoo colors and skin pigmentation, and overall capabilities. All lasers were not created equally, and there remains significant disagreements regarding the best laser for a particular tattooed person (considering skin color, tattoo color(s), healing ability, and final result). A laser for hair removal is best at that and cannot do fat liquefaction or laser eye surgery. Just "having a laser" is not sufficient information. Modern lasers are specifically made for one or two uses (example: tattoo removal and scar treatments). Tattoo removal lasers are created and refined for that task.

The general consensus in the medical world is the Q-switched Neodymium-YAG Laser (Nd:YAG Laser) and the Q-switched Alexandrite Laser are the best for tattoo removal. Your best bet will always be to find someone with a specialized 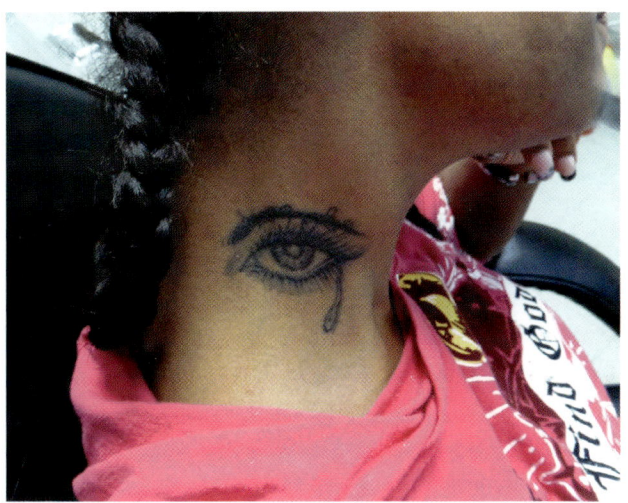 laser refined for the colors in your tattoo, and then determine if that particular laser is also right for your skin color/pigmentation.

The vast majority of tattoo removal lasers were designed for, and therefore work best in, lighter skin tones. The laser focuses on the color of the ink and is "confused" by similar colors in a person's skin. The standard tattoo-removing laser will work best with black, blue, and dark green, and not as effective with orange or yellows. The development of tattoo removal machines refined for darker-skinned individuals has lagged significantly behind that for the lighter skinned. As more people request tattoo removal, the industry will respond with a wider range of more selectively precise lasers.

Once you've found a competent laser tattoo removal specialist, there are a few basics you must understand. Healthy skin will lead to a healthy recovery. Good nutrition and a healthy diet will lead to faster healing. Any type of infection brewing, or recent skin infection recovery, especially Herpes infections, should prompt you to re-schedule your appointment after a full resolution of the symptoms. Also remember to mention any history of keloid formation or abnormal healing as this may occur after the procedure and not help the outcome at all.

Amateur/prison/house party tattoos can usually be removed after 5 to 10 sessions in one- to two-month intervals. Professional tattoos and those with heavy metals in their ink are usually more resistant and may require as many as 20 visits! Be patient.

Watch out for post-laser complications, and work to prevent them. Continue to keep the location clean and moisturized, alert your doctor if an infection develops, and finally. . . don't pick with it!

Chemical Treatments

Another very popular way to attempt to remove a tattoo is to chemically burn it off with acids or bases. Sometimes called a chemical peel, this can be effective in certain 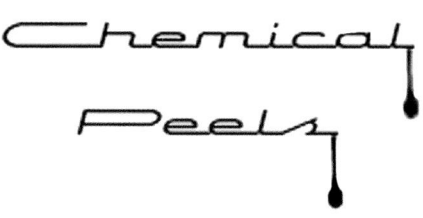 cases where the tattoo is somewhat faded. Like laser removal, this technique works better in amateur, prison, or house party tattoos. By using an acid or strong base, the tattoo is essentially repeatedly burned off until no pigment remains. Scarring is common with this approach but some people prefer the scar to whomever's name was there!

Cut the tattoo out

For years surgeons have known how to either cut a tattoo out or deeply scrape a tattoo off. A small tattoo can simply be cut out, and the two sides can be 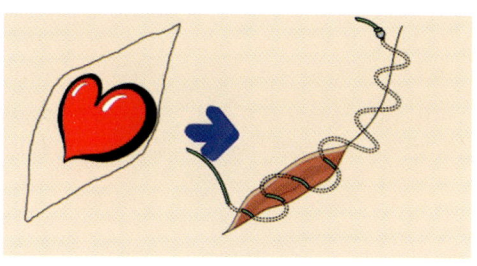 sewn back together as in the picture here. The tattoo can also be shaved off with a thin blade and the area left to heal -- or skin from another area can be transplanted. Scarring is common.

Sand it off

There have been a number of attempts to simply sand or rub the tattoo and the overlying skin off. This is painful, can result in scarring, and is now simply too barbaric to endorse. People have used a salt mix and simply rubbed violently but have found that: 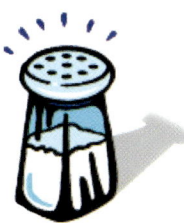 (1) it doesn't work (tattoo pigment remains) and (2) it leaves an ugly scar, and in many cases the old tattoo was preferable. Definitely don't try this at home.

Miracle Lotions and Fading creams

Unfortunately, for most people, fading creams and lotions don't work. If you see an advertisement, please read the fine print, and look for the disclaimer "results in photo not typical." The creams that actually were successful to a

Results *NOT* Typical

degree were found to cause serious health problems in some people. Remember that there is no easy way to remove a tattoo. That's the whole point of a tattoo being permanent. If anyone promises a simple solution to tattoo removal, be very suspicious.

Cover it with another tattoo

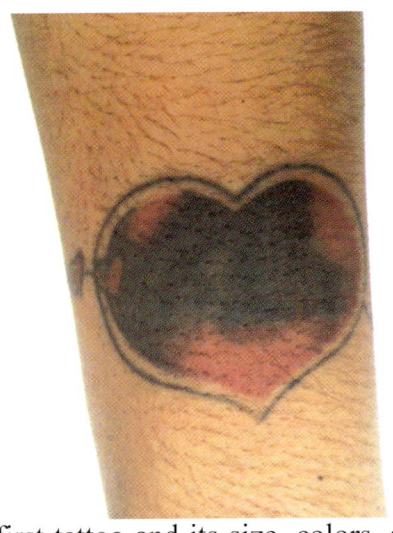

Although this is technically not a removal procedure, the majority of people not happy with a tattoo take the economical approach and attempt to cover the first tattoo with another hopefully more pleasing one. This choice is the easiest because it is cheaper to pay for another tattoo than to pay for multiple visits and treatments involved in tattoo removal. Obviously, the final result depends on the first tattoo and its size, colors, and boldness. Also crucial is the tattoo artist, as the level of expertise needed to successfully cover another tattoo is high. Covering one tattoo with another only helps people who like tattoos and don't mind a larger and more obvious one replacing the first. The best technique for cover-up tattoos involves losing the first tattoo in the design of a second tattoo and changing the focal point of the tattoo to a different region. For this reason the tattoo must be significantly larger and much more complex.

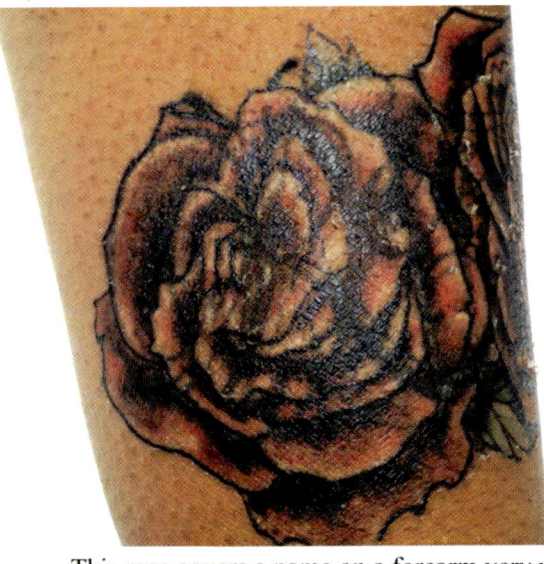

The ultimate irony for some tattoo cover-up recipients is that they continue to "see" the

This rose covers a name on a forearm very well.

original tattoo just as clearly as before. While others only see the new design, the tattoo owner is still "haunted" by that lost lover's name or the botched original tattoo. By far the majority of tattoo cover-ups involve names, so burying letters in a design is no easy task. The best approach is to avoid names and letters altogether.

The bands below the roses hide five large letters, and this person continues to see those letters -- and that name -- every time she looks at her forearm.

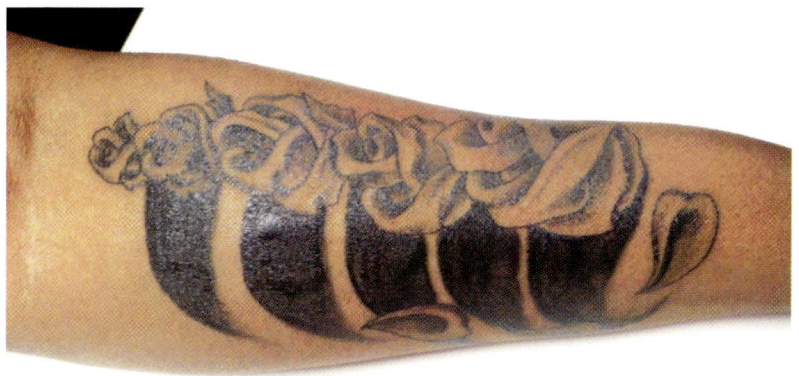

Summary

    Whatever removal or cover-up process you choose, the absolute best option is to get a tattoo after deliberate thought, intense research, and reflection . . . or to not get one at all.

"After getting the 'love of my life's' name tattooed across my lower back, we had a fight and he left. I didn't have the money for tattoo removal, or the energy to think of something bigger to cover the now hated name. So I had the guy down the street just tattoo over it . . . anything so I didn't have to see this huge mistake. As bad as this looks, I prefer it over the name"

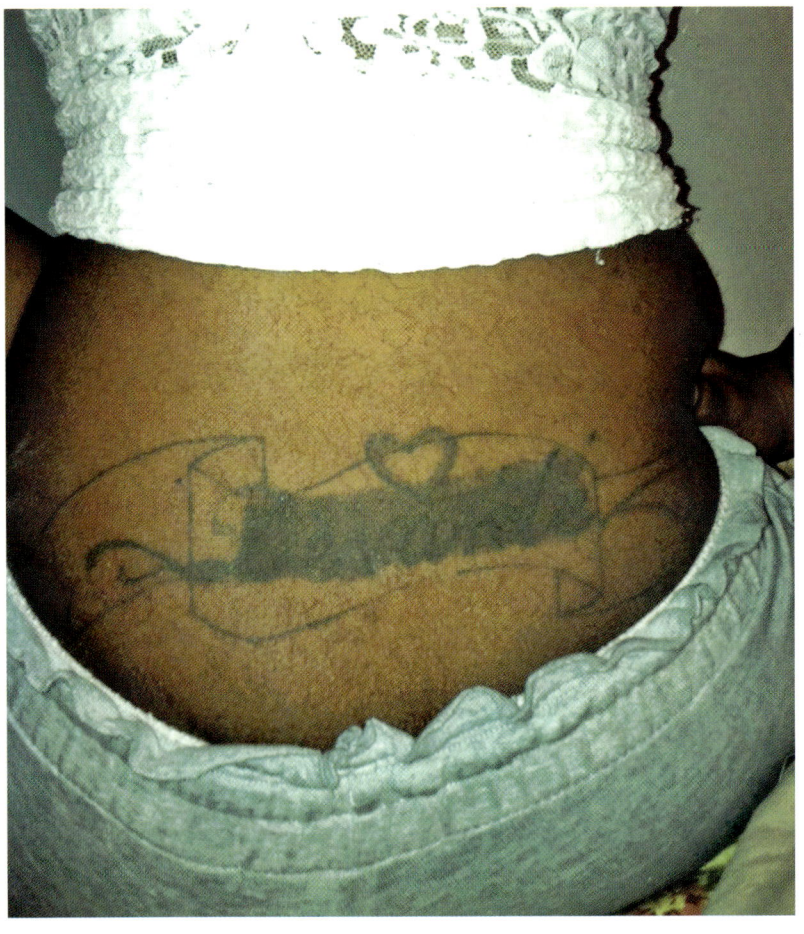

Chapter 10: The PIERCING Truth

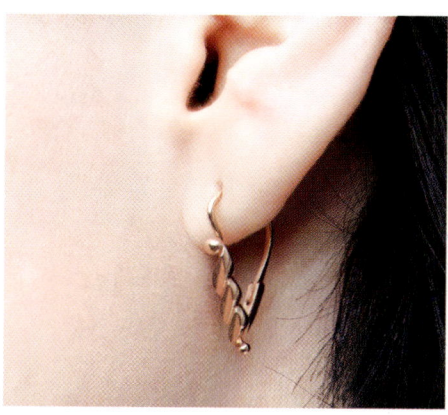

Close on the heels of tattoos in increased popularity is the number of people getting body piercing. Eighty percent of women get their earlobes pierced, and this custom enjoys complete social and medical acceptance. The ear lobe is a relatively safe location of the body to pierce because it has no muscle, cartilage, or much in the way of nerves to damage. The history of ear piercing goes back to the beginnings of human time, and while some people do have complications, by and large, most people have no medical or social problems resulting from having their earlobes pierced.

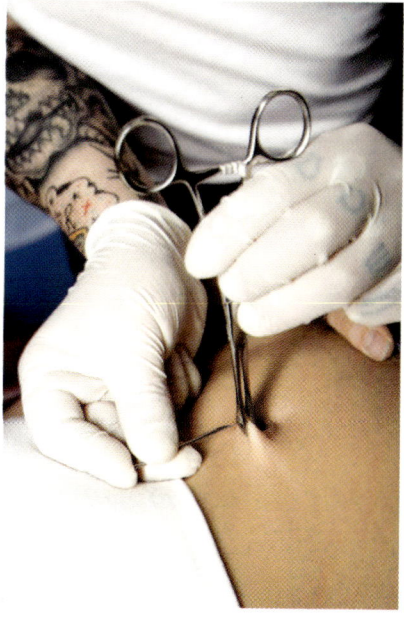

Outside of ear lobe piercing, there has been an explosion in the number and location of body piercing elsewhere. A staggering 25% of all women are getting pierced body parts (other than earlobes). One in ten men are also getting pierced and placing various forms of jewelry. With

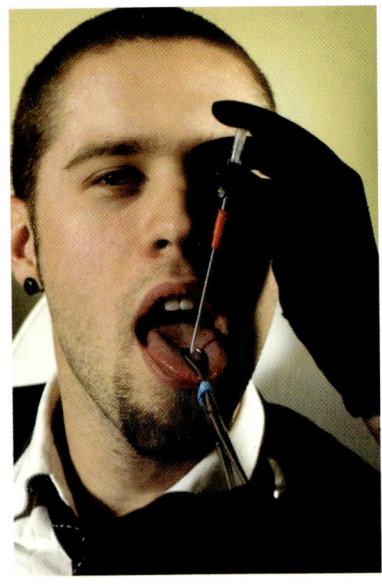

women, this trend began with getting a second piercing in the ear lobe higher, and as time progressed, earrings were placed around the entire circumference of the ear. The next most popular location for body piercing in girls is the navel (belly button), while for men a tongue piercing is the second most common location after the ear. Both sexes can be found with nose piercings, but women lead the pack. In all, people have pierced practically all external locations on the body, and unfortunately, some internal locations as well!

If done safely and by a trained professional, piercing can be a perfectly acceptable way of adorning the body. But in untrained hands, body piercing can lead to months of pain and possibly years of suffering.

Doctors and nurses spend many years learning the human anatomy. They learn where the nerves and arteries are, as well as where they are not. Knowing where a nerve or artery "is not" allows you to avoid these critical structures during a piercing. Many people

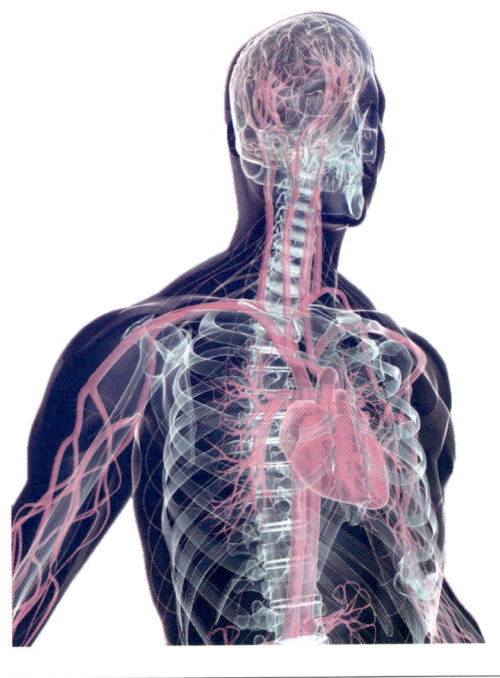

report permanent nerve damage or prolonged bleeding when piercing unconventional locations and hitting and injuring vital nerves or arteries. Research about the risks of getting a piercing in a particular location of the body is a very important step BEFORE you get a piercing.

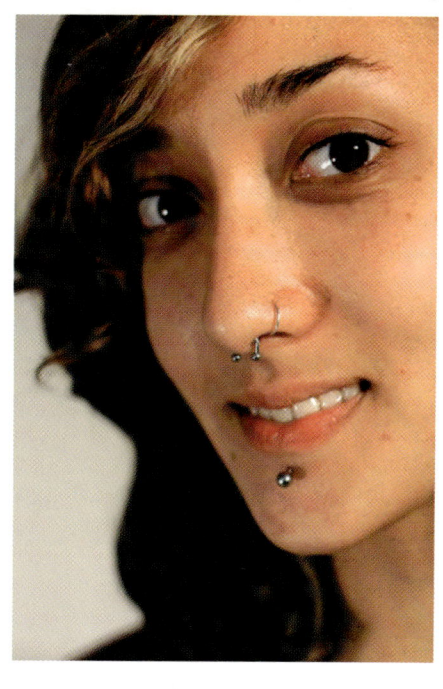

Emergency rooms frequently see infections from poorly sterilized skin and piercing equipment, boils developing, and disfiguring scars from poorly trained piercers. It is important to note that dermatologists (doctors that specialize in diseases of the skin) frown on piercing any location other than the ear lobe mainly because of the damage that can be done to muscles, arteries, nerves, and cartilage.

The tongue, cheek, and mouth piercings are universally rejected by dentists because having all or part of the jewelry in the mouth causes chronic infections that lead to halitosis (bad breath), tooth injury, and pre-mature decay. The overwhelming urge to "play with" the jewelry with your tongue leads to prolonged healing, smoldering infection, and enlarging of the pierced hole.

There is a great increase in antibiotic-resistant bacteria in the community, and as infections progress faster, there are some instances where life-threatening situations occur. Bacteria and viruses can easily be transmitted during piercing and -- because of the depth of some piercing -- can even travel throughout the body, causing system-wide disease. Piercing should be performed by trained professionals in a clean and sterile environment. While it is hard to mess up an earlobe piercing, it is

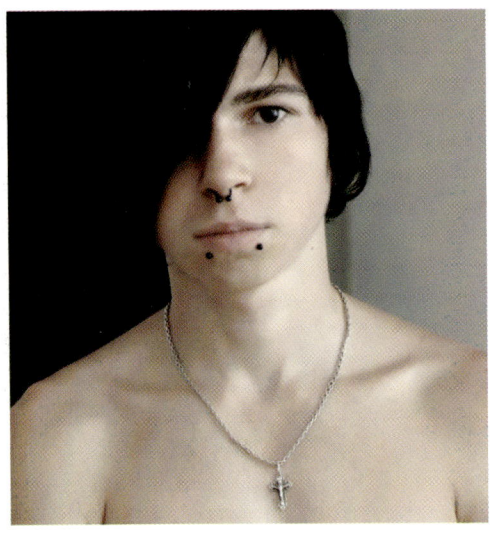

difficult to safely pierce other areas. It is NOT just a matter of sticking a needle through skin.

Even if you get your piercing by a trained professional, healing time for various locations is startlingly long. Piercing in the mouth or private genital areas can take a year or longer to completely heal! A nose or eyebrow piercing could take 6 to 8 weeks to heal, and if you change your mind, they almost always leaves a small yet noticeable scar or skin defect. A skin reaction called "contact dermatitis" can appear as a reaction from less expensive jewelry and if untreated can lead to permanent scaring.

It is very important to learn about every aspect of body piercing BEFORE you dive into something that may have a lifelong effect.

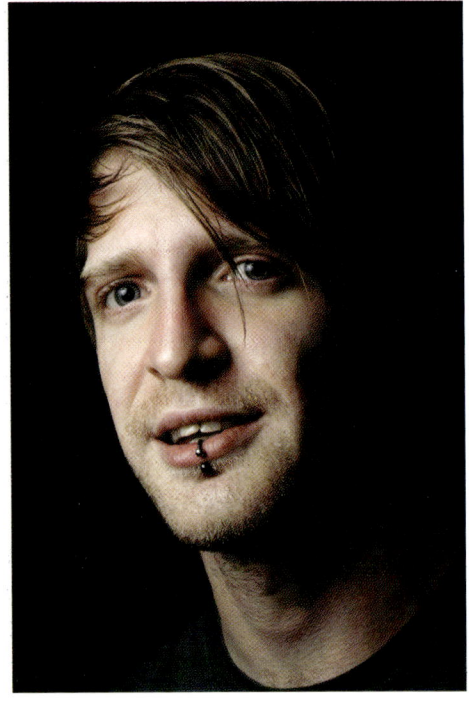

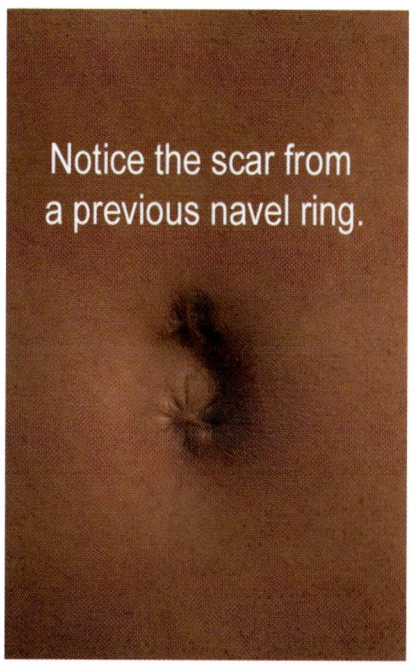

Notice the scar from a previous navel ring.

School is not the place to get a body piercing.

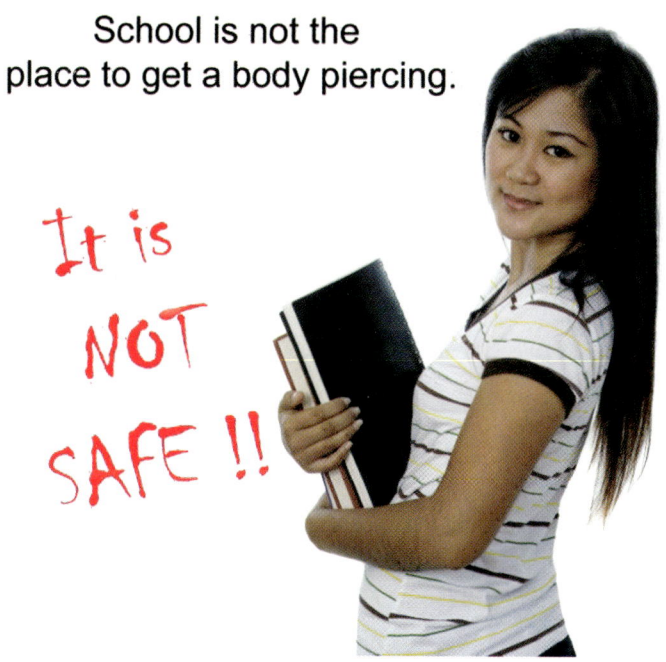

It is NOT SAFE !!

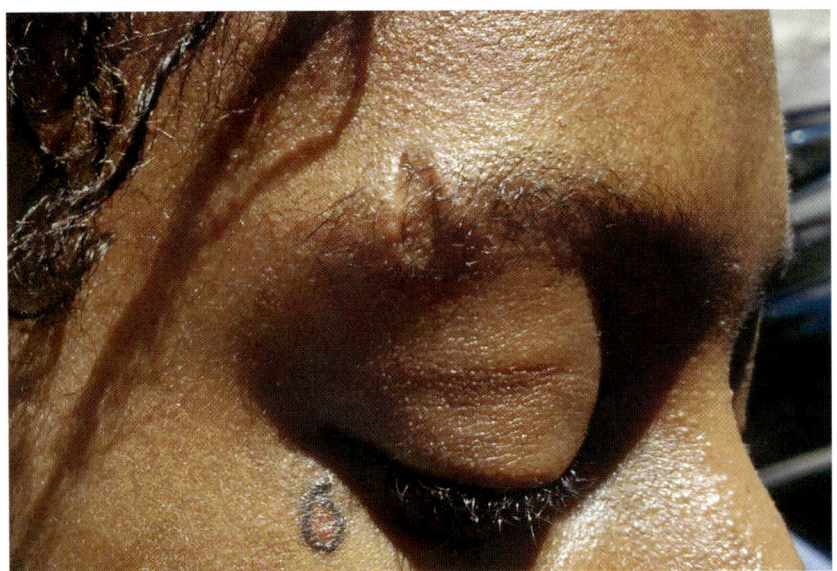

Her baby accidently ripped out her eyebrow piercing.
This is the scar left behind.

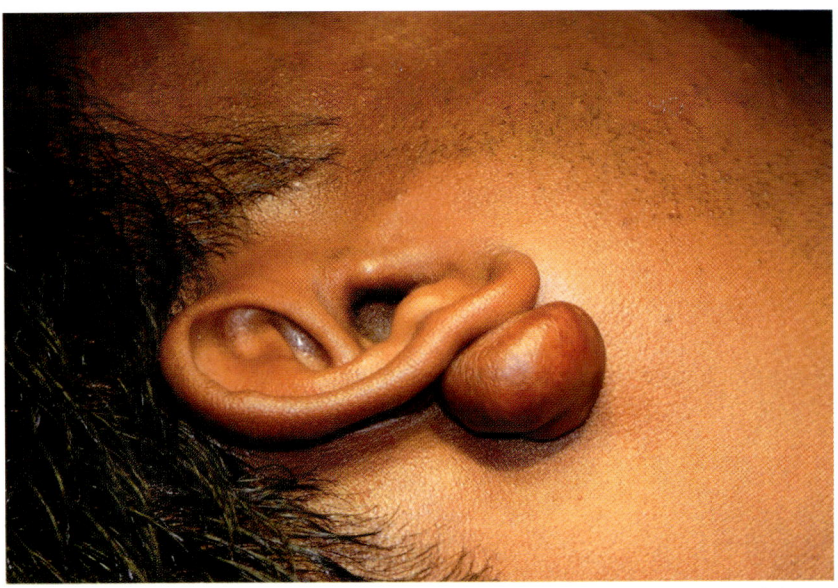

Even a simple ear piercing can cause problems if not done safely

Chapter 11: Body Art and Your Future

The tattoo craze will end, but tattoos and piercings will most definitely continue; the history of human-kind has borne that out. There are many individuals that consider their tattoo a part of their personae. These people are the natural recipients of tattoos;

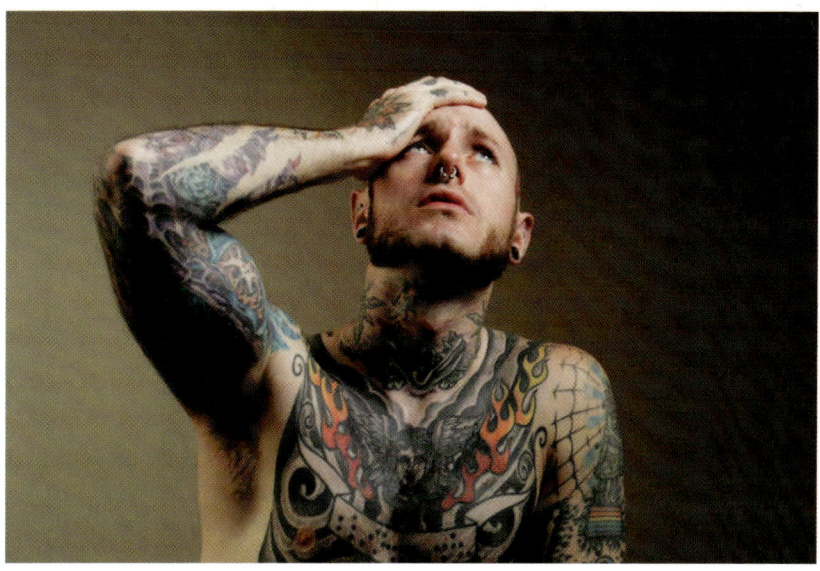

they are the population that would always get body art, whether it was a fad or not. They have no regrets or remorse over their tattoo: It is part of who they are. Most others, modern fad aside, would not even think of tattoos; it would not be on their radar screen of interests.   These carefree tattoo adopters end up regretting their decision somewhere down the road, mainly because they didn't research the topic, think long and hard enough about it, and reflect on their own personality and goals -- in addition to insuring that the location, tattooist, and art was appropriate for their body. This book is for that second group.

The human body is a beautiful creation in all of its shapes, sizes, and colors. If a permanent mark is to be placed on the body for the rest of its life, think about the consequences, your personality, your future, your goals, your children, and your other regrets in life so far. The data supports the fact that a majority of people getting a tattoo today will hide it, camouflage it, remove it, or regret it before the end of their life. That may not be everybody -- but it is indeed most of those who have tattoos.

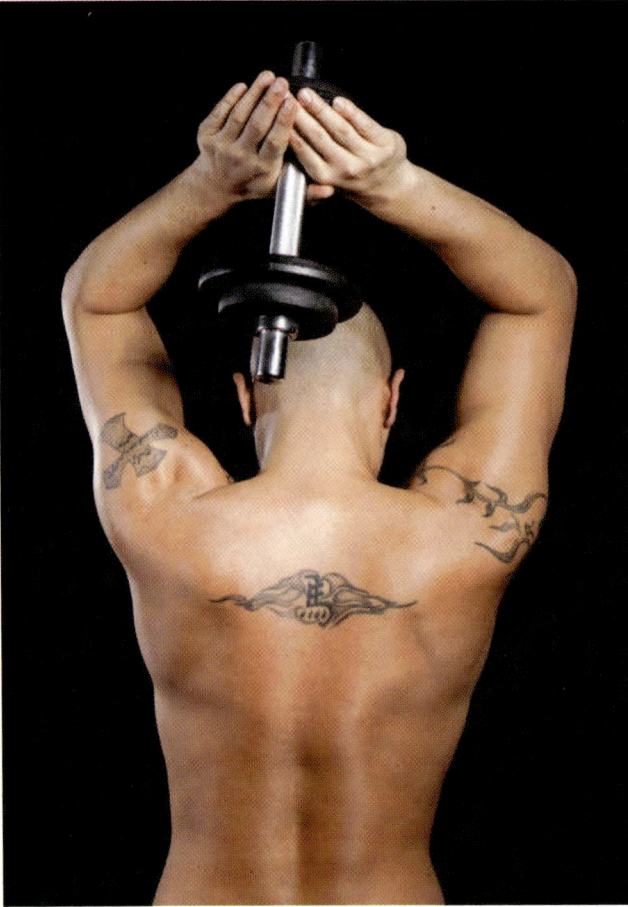

Fads, like getting tattoos and piercings, will fade and be replaced by something newer. The old trends will be replaced by new trends. Body art has always been an aspect of human culture and -- as advances occur -- new forms of body art will take their position in society.

People will be able to guess your age based on the design, content, number, and location of your tattoos.

Imagine the conversation in the year 2025. . . "Look at the poor woman. . .she thought she was cute back in 2012, and she looks so stupid now! I bet she wishes that thing could come off. Her tattoo says 'Hot Mamma'. . .maybe back then she was, but that certainly

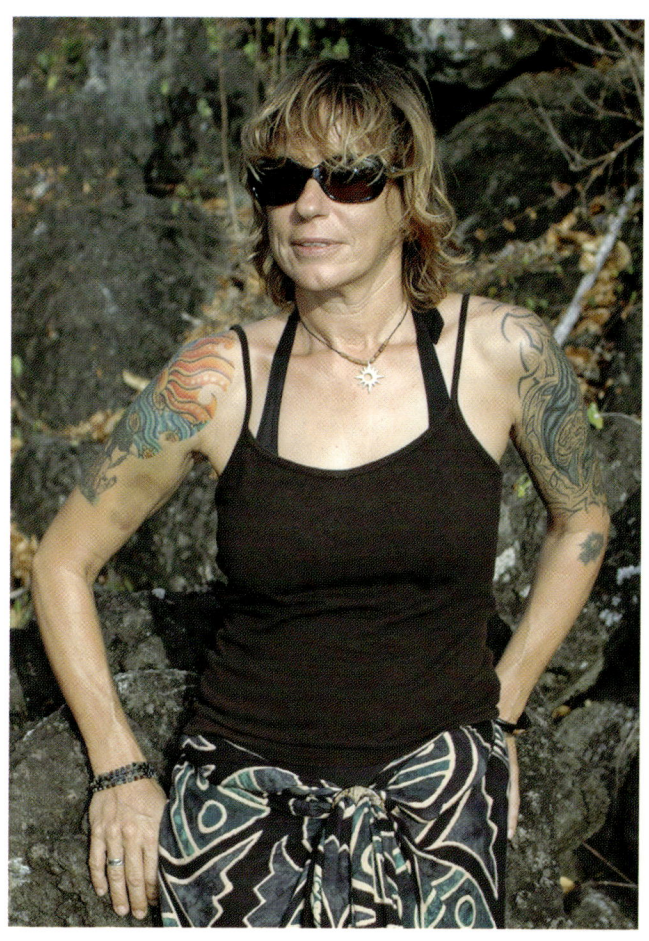

does not describe her now. Now her 12-year-old daughter says she wants to be a 'hot mamma' too!"

The simple fact is teens and young adults are acquiring tattoos younger, faster, and repeatedly without adequate thought. Some will be comfortable with their tattoos the rest of their lives. Others will cringe every time they see it because it is a painful reminder of a youthful ignorance, a lost love, or a drunken indiscretion. The key to avoiding these regrets is to instill a sense of urgency and permanence to the act of tattooing or piercing. Today's young people should consider tattooing or piercing to be the big decision that it is. High school students are secretly getting tattoos and piercings across the country without parental approval or permission. College students are getting tattoos at parties and in dorm rooms as a result of peer pressure and the wish to make a BIG decision about their life. Neither group is really getting all the information they need to make a good decision. Psychologists have found that those that think long and hard about a decision tend to not regret it down the road.

New Inks and Body Art of the Future

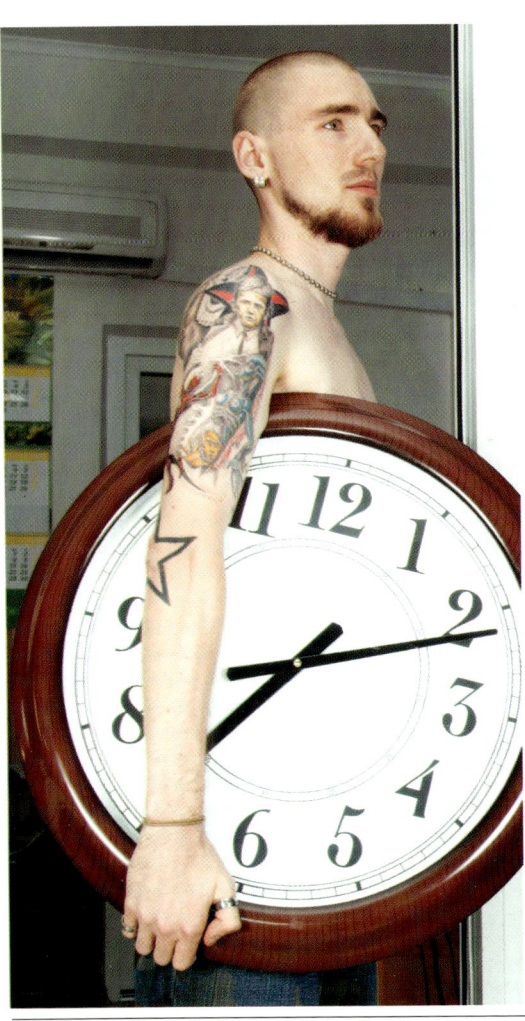

Advancements in ink, application, and semi-permanent tattoos are being developed. More recently, a company has developed a dye that is "not necessarily permanent." The dye can be removed by a specialized laser more easily and with fewer treatments at whatever time the person chooses. Critics question whether consumers would adopt non-permanent tattoo ink -- since the permanency of it is the whole point. If a person thought enough to get removable ink when getting a tattoo, he or she would probably not get one in the first place.

It is likely that 10 years from now, vivid and colorful semi-permanent (lasting six months to a year) ink could be available for tattoo artists to use and re-use. People might also still complain that they have to look at a temporary tattoo for too long. *Imagine being saddled with one forever.*

The body art of the future will be more flexible. Art will be camouflaged during the workday and in full effect at night when you're on the town. It can be nicely hidden when on a job interview, and then flashed on a beach. And the best part will be your ability to change your mind.

Give the decision to get a tattoo or piercing the consideration it warrants. It's a big move, and one that will be with you the rest of your life. Your life, your loves, your children, and your family and friends will all be affected by your decision to get body art. Consider the health risks, the artist, the design, the size, and your future. If you give this decision the time and energy it deserves, there is no question you will be happy with your final choice.

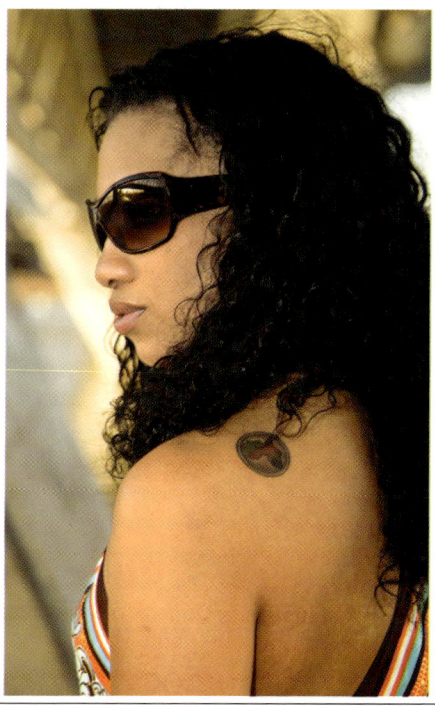

About the Author

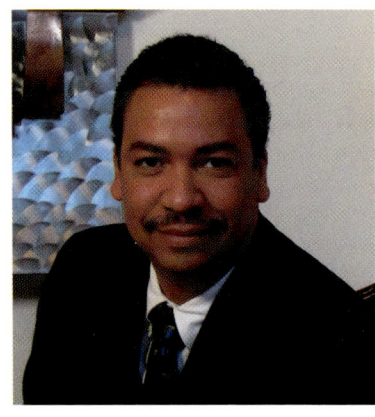

Gregory L. Hall, MD, is a primary care physician practicing in Cleveland, Ohio for the past 20 years. He has lectured on various topics ranging from hypertension to alternative medicine, but his latest passion is to improve the general public's knowledge about the societal, health, and psychological impact of permanent body art.

After graduation from Williams College with a bachelor's degree in psychology, he attended the Medical College of Ohio, and completed residency in internal medicine at the Cleveland Clinic.

Dr. Hall serves on the teaching faculty at Case Western Reserve University's College of Medicine and has an appointment of assistant professor. He has co-chaired the City of Cleveland's Public Health Advisory Committee, and co-chaired the leadership board of *Steps to a Healthier Cleveland* which oversaw health awareness and improvement activities throughout the area. In 2002, Dr. Hall received a governor's appointment to the Ohio Commission on Minority Health, on which he now serves as Chairman. In January of 2008, he was appointed to Ohio Medicaid's Health Advisory Board and served on its Executive Committee. In 2010, he was appointed to the Cuyahoga County Board of Health which oversees Ohio's largest county's broad range of quality driven public health programs and services.